YOU WONDERFUL BOY

YOU WONDERFUL BOY

A mother's bond with her son through his severe OCD, addiction, and his death.

Jennifer Liberatore

NFB Publishing
Buffalo, New York

You Wonderful Boy: A mother's bond with her son through his severe OCD, addiction , and his death./ Liberatore 1st Edition

ISBN: 978-1-953610-76-8

Nonfiction> Memoir
Nonfiction> Family Dynamic> Addiction
Nonfiction> Mental Health> OCD
Nonfiction> Eating Disorders
Nonfiction> Biography
Nonfiction>Social Issue
Nonfiction> Loss of a Child> Bereaved Parent
Nonfiction> Grief

Cover Design By Hannah Taylor (ahollowbone.com)

Please contact ahollowbone.com for more information

NFB Publishing
119 Dorchester Road
Buffalo, New York 14213
For more information visit Nfbpublishing.com

This book is dedicated to my four sons, the lights of my life, my greatest blessings.

To Christopher, Eric and Peter, who by their very existence, carried me through the darkest time of my life.

And to Zach, who taught me to be brave.

INTRODUCTION

"I carry your heart (I carry it in my heart)"
- E.E. Cummings

On October 2nd, 2020, my son Zach died. My beautiful boy, my first born son, my Zach-a-doo crossed over to the other side. Even writing those words feels inherently wrong, surreal. It's now three years later and it still feels like it can't possibly be true. My life was forever changed. There are no words in the English language to describe the pain of losing a child; tragic, heartbreaking, devastating, are words that don't even come close to describing the gaping hole left inside your heart. I have always compared having a child to a scene in Dr. Seuss's *The Grinch*; when the Grinch's heart grows from a tiny speck, to so big that it's barely contained in his body. That's how if felt to me when Zach was born, like my heart would explode, and every child I had expanded that love even more. I suppose that's why it hurts deeper than anything in life when that giant heart is shattered. I felt like I had lost a piece of my soul.

If you are reading this and you've lost a child, I am so deeply sorry. I wish I could shield every parent from having to go through this unimaginable pain. When Zach died, I began hearing an expression from other parents who had lost a child: "You've joined a club that you never wanted to join." No truer words, but in my experience, this club can help to heal your pain. In any situation in life, whether it be grief, trauma, mental illness, or addiction, hearing another person's similar story resonates with you, helping you to feel less isolated.

I am writing this book for several reasons. For a very long time, I thought that Zach and I would someday write a book together. Zach died of an overdose, but it was mental illness that killed him. I was sure that he would someday overcome his severe obsessive-compulsive disorder, anxiety disorders, and addiction, and that we would write a book together to help others. He was a beautiful and gifted writer. After he died, I soon realized that we would still write a book together, with him on the other side. While he was alive, Zach was an advocate for mental illness and addiction, bringing awareness and breaking the stigma. I feel that it's my job to continue that legacy.

I am writing this book to tell my Zach's story, to keep his memory alive, and because I feel that it's an important story to tell. If you are someone who is struggling with mental illness or addiction, or you have a loved one who does, I hope that hearing our story helps you feel less alone. I know that's what Zach has always wanted.

I also want to share my experience with Zach on the other side; to relay all of the incredible signs and messages he has sent us to let us know he is not really "gone." He is always with us, and he is doing amazing things from the other side.

Finally, I write this to tell my story of how I pulled myself out of the darkness and into the light. It is my hope that hearing about my journey of self healing will help you in some way.

PART 1

My Story

"Two roads diverged in a wood, and I - I took the one less traveled by,
and that has made all the difference."
- Robert Frost

CHAPTER ONE

I START WITH MY story because in the many nonfiction books I've read in my life, I've always personally liked to hear the author's story. Also, I will be talking about my spiritual views in this book, and I'd like to share all of the events and soul searching that led me to the place where I am now.

I was born in Buffalo, New York, and grew up in Hamburg, a suburb south of Buffalo. I was the oldest of three children (brother Peter and sister Kerry) born to my parents Constance and Richard. The one thing that I always knew to be true in this life is how much my parents loved us. We grew up in a small, charming house in a neighborhood where we played kickball in the court and rode our bikes to the playground. There were times that our family struggled financially, but my parents always provided us with the best life possible.

We had our challenges, as all families do. My dad battled alcoholism throughout my entire childhood. Addiction would become a theme in my life. He was in and out of rehab facilities a couple of times during my teen years, but by the time I turned 18, he became sober and continued to stay sober for the rest of his life. He was always my hero for that. My dad was, quite simply, the best man I have ever known. He was the kindest, most honest, genuine, hard working, altruistic soul. He never cared for material things. His only goal in life was just to take care of his family, and that he did. He adored my mom. We were his pride and joy, along with our home. He was a sheet metal worker at the Ford Motor plant for most of his life, and he could build anything in our house, and fix anything. He called me "Muffin" (short for blueberry muffin).

While I was growing up, my mom was always a pillar of strength for our family, holding it together through hard times. She was beautiful, smart, strong, independent, outgoing, and kind. She was a classic Leo - she could chat with anyone, and loved a good party. She loved hosting cookouts and holiday dinners at our house. She was an X-ray technician, working in the emergency room at Buffalo Mercy Hospital when we were young, and later on in a private office. I learned my best qualities from my mom: strength, independence, and compassion. Her favorite saying was, "But for the grace of God, go I." She was always donating items to food pantries, and money to any charity that sent her a letter.

I adored my brother and sister, even though at times we fought, as many children do. The two of them were always very close growing up, with similar interests, especially music. They were cool and fun, but my interests were always very different from theirs, until we became adults. The three of us are quite close now and my sister Kerry is one of my best friends.

In my life, I have always felt like I didn't quite fit in, and I suppose that began with my family. As a very young child, I can remember being able to see "spirits" and angels, but I was not allowed to talk about it in a Catholic family or at school, and so I stopped seeing them. I remember feeling extremely alone when I stopped seeing them.

The things that I loved most in my childhood were school, dance, and books, not necessarily in that order. I loved school. I loved learning and writing and reading. Schoolwork always came easily to me, and I always excelled academically. I suppose we like the things that we are good at. When I wasn't at school, I had my head buried in a book, or I was at dance. I began dance lessons at 3 and by 12 years old, I was taking ballet lessons six days a week and performing regularly. At 16, I auditioned for a ballet company in the city of Buffalo, called Buffalo Ballet Theatre. Every day after school, I had to take two metro buses to get there, but I didn't care. I loved every minute. Dance was one of the loves of my life, and I finally found somewhere where I felt like I fit in.

My parents were devout Catholics and we were raised as such. I attended public schools through ninth grade and then switched over to Immaculata Academy, an all girl Catholic high school. This transpired because my best friend Renee talked me into it. My mom was thrilled. (Renee later switched back to our former school, so we lost touch for awhile, but we are still friends today.) I have always believed that everything happens for a reason, though we may never know what that reason is. Looking back, that switch to Immaculata would bring me to the next chapter of my life. It's as though my spirit guides orchestrated the whole thing. (I am sure they did.)

Switching schools is how I would meet Sue, my best friend for life. I still clearly remember the day she came over to my house to welcome me to my new school and my head was buried in a book. Her family became a second family to me. Her older brothers and sisters are like the older siblings I never had. They have always been there for me, even to this day. Susie would bring fun into my serious high school life of schoolwork and ballet. She helped me feel more connected at school and introduced me to friends and parties in our neighborhood. Forty years later, she is still my BFF and in this life, she is one of the people who always has my back; she always believes in me. She even encouraged me to write after Zach died, which motivated me to write this book. I am so grateful for her beautiful soul in my life.

Sue talked me into joining CYO (Catholic Youth Organization), which was basically social events with kids from several schools. It was there that I would meet Peter, my future husband, and father of our four sons. Truth be told, he kicked a ball across the gym and it hit me in the face and that is how we met. It's not a surprising "meet cute" given that our life would later revolve around basketballs and footballs. (I should have seen the foreshadowing there.) He was handsome, kind, smart, and funny. He was the fun to my serious and the outgoing to my quiet. We were high school sweethearts and would get married nine years later.

First came New York City. As much as I loved school, and knew that I would someday go to college, I wanted to dance first. Dance brought me so much joy, especially performing. It was my passion. I lived and breathed dance, and always felt like I was "home" on stage. So while all of my classmates were going off to college, I moved to New York City to go to the Joffrey Ballet School. I was 18 years old. My parents must have been terrified, but they let me go. I suppose they couldn't have stopped me if they tried. I found a waitressing job within a week and lived at Swiss House, a residence for girls on the Upper West Side. I would dance for four hours during the day and then work in the restaurant for seven hours at night. It was exhausting, even for an 18 year old. That physically exhausting pace caught up with me and I left Joffrey. I continued to take classes and worked at several restaurants over the years, where I would meet some of my lifelong friends. I lived at a couple of different apartments over the years, living in Hell's Kitchen for the most part. Though trendy now, back in the 80's, it was an inexpensive place to live and consisted mainly of theatre people. My roommates became like family to me.

Over the course of the next few years, I landed a job with a ballet company in Connecticut, performed with my friend Michelle's modern company, and did some modeling type jobs, such as appearing on a couple of MTV specials with Alan Hunter, which was really fun. In the winter of 1987, I suffered a pretty bad knee injury while ice skating at Rockefeller Center. The injury and the high cost of living wore on me, and Peter and my family were in Buffalo, so I decided it was time to move back to Buffalo and go to college. I was only in New York for three years, but it felt like ten. I had so many invaluable experiences and friendships, and I grew up quickly, living on my own. It was an important chapter, and I will always be grateful for that time in my life.

In the fall of 1987, I became a student at UB, the State University of New York at Buffalo. The first week of school, I met my friend Lynn who talked me into auditioning for Zodiaque, the resident dance company. So even though my major was psychology, I spent most of my time in the dance department, taking classes and performing with Zodiaque, again, where I felt like I fit in. The teachers and dancers became like family to me over the course of my time at UB. My good friend Lisa, who I had met in New York, came to UB to dance and we became roommates. For the next four years that was my life: college, dance, work, hanging out with Lisa and my dance friends, and Peter.

I had fully intended on going to graduate school to become a psychologist or mental health counselor, but life got in the way. I had the opportunity to dance with a local ballet company called Buffalo City Ballet, as well as other performing opportunities, so I continued to dance, while working as the aerobics and fitness director of the McKinley Park Health Club which was owned by Peter's father. I've literally been teaching exercise my whole life, beginning with ballet and aerobics when I was 16.

I graduated from UB with a B.A. in psychology in the spring of 1991, and Peter and I were married in June of 1992. The wedding was a happy time for our families. My mom and I spent a lot of time on the wedding plans with Peter's mom, Mary. She was like a second mom to me, and she would become one of my best friends. I continued performing and working, while Peter worked for his dad's company, as well as starting his own company, and we built a beautiful home to start a family in. Life was good.

CHAPTER TWO

ZACHARY PETER LIBERATORE was born on December 19th, 1995. He was born with a thick head of dark hair and dark Italian skin. He was perfect in our eyes. He was our everything, a dream come true. He was the first grandchild and nephew on both sides of our family, so to say he was adored is an understatement. For me, it felt like my new life began, my life as a mom. From the moment I saw him, I felt like I'd known him forever. I would stare at his beautiful face for hours. I vowed to be the best mom I possibly could. I vowed to protect him.

We were typical of our generation of parenting. We read all of the parenting books, bought the safest car seat, researched the best stroller, worried about him when he had a cold, made sure he ate enough vegetable baby food, and read him stories every night. The baby nursery was decorated with carousel horses with a white sleigh crib. He was colicky for a couple months, so I spent hours dancing with him and rocking him in the nursery. Besides the colic, he was an easy baby, sleeping through the night at a young age. I called him "Zach-a-doo." His dad called him "Doo." We were so happy with our beautiful boy.

For the next two and a half years, Zachary and I would always be together. He was such an easy child. Even as a toddler, he had a zen nature. I would take him to a playgroup (as first time mothers often do) and when the other kids took toys from him, he would just smile at them. I worried that he would get stepped on in life, but I later realized that was just his nature. Even then, he knew what was important and what wasn't. He was so chill for a toddler. There was no "terrible twos" period with him. He would sit in a high chair for hours at a restaurant, just eating and smiling. He was a beautiful boy with thick, wavy hair, big brown eyes that sparkled, and a smile that would light up a room.

He loved animals, especially elephants. He always had a small toy animal in his hand. We would often take him to the zoo and he would just stand in front of the elephants, watching them. Something about their gentle nature has always reminded me of Zach. He loved *The Lion King* movie, we watched it hundreds of times. I can still hear him singing *Circle of Life*. Like all kids born in the 90's, he loved Barney the purple dinosaur. I think I knew the words to every Barney song. His very favorite character was Disney's "Pluto" doggie and carried him around for years. He chewed on the nose so much, I had to sew it back on at least ten times.

His dad always said that he was a big mama's boy (this is true). He did struggle with separation anxiety when he was young. When I would drop him off at pre school, he would stand in the doorway, silently watching me leave and would take awhile to acclimate to the class every day. It always tugged at my heartstrings, but he would eventually have fun. I would learn many years later that extreme OCD patients often had separation anxiety when they were young.

Two and a half years after Zach was born, in June 1998, our son Christopher was born. My heart expanded even more. When Peter brought Zach to the hospital to meet his new baby brother, I put my arms out for him to come to me because we had never been separated for that long. He went right past me to his new brother, arms outstretched, his chubby hands shaking in anticipation of holding Christopher. And so it began ... he was born to be a big brother. One of our first photos of Christopher is of Zach holding him protectively, beaming with pride and love.

While Zach looked like his dad, but had my quiet, serious, introspective personality, Christopher was the polar opposite. He looked more like my family with his fair skin and light eyes, but his personality was just like his dad; outgoing, fun, charming, energetic, funny. Zach adored him, as we all did. I called him Christopher Robin since he loved Winnie the Pooh. The two of them were best friends and partners in crime. Christopher helped to bring Zach out of his shell with his fearless, outgoing nature. One of my favorite memories of the two of them took place at a friend's birthday party. There was a DJ playing music and a couple people were dancing. Christopher was one of them. He was not even 2 yrs old and he was out on the dance floor, uninhibitedly dancing by himself. Zach stood at the edge of the dance floor watching him, with the biggest smile on his face. We looked at each other and laughed. To know Christopher, is to love him.

Our family continued to grow. Our son Eric was born in April 2000, another bright light brought into our lives. When you have children, it's amazing to see that no matter how many children you have, each one is so completely different, completely unique. Eric looked like my sister with his blonde hair and huge green eyes, and he came into our lives like sunshine. In fact, the song I would sing to him as a baby was *Here Comes the Sun* by the Beatles. He has a kind, easy going, gentle nature with a bright smile. His humor has made us laugh for the past 23 years.

Eric adored his big brothers and they became the three musketeers, always laughing, playing, and giggling together. When Eric started talking, he called Zachary "Zachy", Christopher "Toto", and himself "Eekie." The nicknames stuck for many years. Although Eric was always a homebody, preferring to be home with me, he happily tagged along at swim lessons, baseball and soccer. As you may imagine, life was getting crazy with three little boys. Still, I pondered the idea of a fourth baby. I had a miscarriage when Eric was a baby, and then I knew for sure; I was meant to have four children. And so it was.

In September 2002, our son Peter was born, and I cannot imagine my life without him. I had four boys under the age of 6 and life got even crazier. I wouldn't have changed a thing. Peter (or Petes as we called him) is the most positive person I know. He was a bubble of joy from day one. He had huge brown eyes with thick black eyelashes and dimples for days. His laugh was contagious. He is one of those people who comes into a room and makes it brighter; truly a bright light in this world. His enthusiasm for life, (and everything!) is contagious. He rounded out the 4-pack and I have never seen a 4-pack so close. Zach reveled in being their big brother. It was as if he was just waiting for all of them to arrive.

I now look back at that time of my life of being newly married, and having babies, as my "Camelot." It seemed too good to be true. I had four beautiful, healthy children and I loved being a mom more than anything in the world. Our wedding and our sons brought our families even closer. Peter's parents lived across the street from us and our families often got together for dinners and birthdays. My brother Peter has lived out of state since his 20's, but our parents, and my sister Kerry, and Peter's sister Carol spent a lot of time together, usually revolving around my boys. The two aunts didn't have kids of their own; they adored their nephews and they were a huge part of my sons' lives. One of the things that has always brought me the most joy is having family at my house for holidays and birthdays.

We live in a town just south of Buffalo, called Orchard Park. If you are a football fan, you know that this is the home of the Buffalo Bills stadium, sacred ground in our family. My boys were all sports obsessed like their dad; football, baseball, basketball. They did it all. We practically lived at Duerr field, the local baseball park. In the summer, there was typically one game every night, and often three per day on Saturdays and Sundays. Zach and Christopher also played on travel teams, which meant more games even further away. I would be lying if I said I enjoyed baseball games every weekend on glorious summer days, but if I tried to convince the ones who weren't playing to go to a pool, the answer was always no. They loved it. They ran around with their friends eating popsicles and french fries.

The best part of the baseball years for me was meeting my new friends. I met Laura and Debbie when Zach was just 4 yrs old. Their kids and my kids would become the best of friends, as would we. Laura's son Danny was Zach's best friend until the day he died. Christopher, Max and Charlie were the three musketeers, and Eric, Peter, Emily, and Olivia we called "the littles." To this day, we all consider each other to be family. We spent countless hours by my pool while the kids swam, and the boys would always end up on the front lawn playing football, or baseball with a rolled up sock, or some other game we could never quite figure out the rules to. Laura and Debbie were like sisters to me.

I also met my friends Melissa and Stephanie at this time. We were drawn together because we each had four boys. Our twelve boys were all friends and we always had fun gabbing at the endless baseball games. Up until meeting them, all of the women I knew had two boys, or two girls, or a boy and girl. No one I knew had four boys. The three of us have always had fun comparing our crazy boy stories. Life wasn't always easy with four little boys. I was blessed beyond belief, but any mom with small children will tell you that it is physically and emotionally exhausting. My boys rarely fought, but were high energy all the time, literally always moving and wrestling. My mom always asked me why they couldn't just sit and read like I used to (Ha!) Peter and I would take the boys on vacations to Florida and inevitably a woman would look at all of us and ask me, "Are they ALL yours?" Zach would always laugh at that.

Throughout the course of my life, my girlfriends have meant the world to me. I am a girl's girl. The strength and compassion and love from all of these women have gotten me through my most difficult times; my friend Renee in middle school, Sue throughout my whole life, my friends when I lived in NYC, Lisa, Lynn and Beth in college and in dance, and all of my "mom" friends... Laura, Debbie, Melissa, Patty, Christa, Carolyn and too many to name. And then there are my "spiritual friends" Annmarie and Lillian; our discussions over the years ranging from the philosophy of yoga, to angels, to meditation, to fashion. My sister Kerry is my friend, my soul sister, and my confidante. She is my rock, and I don't know how I could have gotten through this life without her. Looking back, I realize

I had assembled an army of incredible women who would help me get through the next chapter of my life. My life was about to become increasingly harder over the next fifteen years.

CHAPTER THREE

Wゝ HEN ERIC WAS a baby, Peter's mom Mary, found out she had breast cancer. She did the chemo and radiation and appeared to be in remission, however a few years later, it came back. It had metastasized in her spine and brain. We watched in horror as her health slowly deteriorated. Cancer is an awful disease. It is often said that people who "beat" cancer are strong, but so are the ones who don't. She was strong and courageous until the end. She died at 65 and nothing would ever be the same for any of us. Her husband had adored her. For Peter, she was the closest person to him in this life and he was devastated. My sons lost their loving, doting "little grandma." It was a huge loss for me as well. She had been a second mom to me for over twenty years, and she was one of my closest friends. She was one of those loving, giving, kind, generous people that everyone loved. She was the glue that held our family together. Unfortunately, after she died, nothing was ever the same.

Soon after that, I found myself in a state of depression. I had never experienced anxiety or depression in my life before, and I didn't know how to handle it, especially with four little boys to take care of. I was raised in an alcoholic family, and I learned later on in counseling that it is common in alcoholic families to not talk about things; problems, feelings, and emotions should be kept to yourself. That was very true for me, and so I didn't talk to anyone about what I was going through, not even my husband or my closest friends. I suffered in silence, although it did not go unnoticed. Whenever I was driving, I was crying, even though I had a 4 yr old in the backseat. I managed to continue taking care of my family: making dinners, doing laundry, and driving to practices and games. But I felt hollow inside and I felt incredibly guilty about that since I had the "perfect" life.

It became increasingly difficult for me to sleep or eat. I had lost a tremendous amount of weight and looked awful. Peter suggested I see a mental health counselor. She ascertained that I was clinically depressed, and suggested that I go on antidepressants.

This was a major turning point in my life, on many levels. I chose not to go on antidepressants because it didn't feel right for me. This is not to say that I don't think it's a good idea for other people to go on medication; it can be very helpful for those who need it. I think that everyone has to follow their own instincts about that. Instead, I wanted to find a way to help myself, to heal myself. Looking back at that time, I now know that I was beginning a spiritual awakening; if only I had known that at the time. Spiritual growth rarely happens when life is good. Spiritual awakenings often come in times of tragedy and personal struggle. They often come in the form of depression, anxiety, and the search for a deeper meaning in life.

I had a wonderful, talented, compassionate mental health counselor who helped me a lot. She happened to be a marriage counselor as well, but unfortunately our marriage couldn't be saved. It had been too many years of hard: Peter's mom's illness and death, and my depression, all the while trying to raise four sons. There was too much of a break to be fixed, and even our boys could feel the tension and sadness. Of course they could. Children feel it all. I obviously want to protect our privacy regarding our divorce, but I will say that the end of our marriage was another death for us to endure. We had been best friends for 24 years, and of course there is tremendous guilt when going through a divorce with children.

The first few years were extremely difficult, but the boys seemed to be doing well. I believe that this was because we maintained the "status quo" for them as much as we could. I stayed in our family home with them and Peter bought a house five minutes away (which was also extremely helpful with all the times that a backpack or baseball glove or football cleats were left at the other house.) They saw their dad every single day. He drove them to school every morning (except high school) and, with our crazy schedule of four boys in sports, we were all together every night and all weekend. It never mattered whose "weekend" it was; we both went to all of their games, all of the time. We continued to celebrate birthdays together, and I still had Peter and his family over for holidays. Maybe that seems a bit odd, but it worked for our family. I am sure that all divorced parents scrutinize their kids for signs of damage. We were no different. Our divorce surely caused my boys pain and for that, I will always be sorry. It brought some comfort that their teachers, coaches and school counselors all reported that they were doing well.

Speaking of school counselors, our family was blessed with the best of them, our Francine. She started babysitting for us when Eric was a two year old, and later tutored Eric and Peter, and is like a member of our family. I don't know what we would have done without her in our lives. She is smart, fun, funny, and one of the most positive, enthusiastic people I know. My sons adore her. Her humor has lifted me out of some really sad moments. She calls herself an "honorary Liberatore," but the honor is all ours; we were blessed to have her watching over our boys. She counseled them without them realizing it, always keeping me updated on how she thought they were all doing. When Francine thought that my sons were all thriving post divorce, I believed it.

I can now say fifteen years later, that the key for us going through divorce with children, was to always put the boys first. This obviously didn't lend well to other relationships, but that is how we chose to do it. Peter was, and is, a stellar dad and my boys are lucky to have him. While there were times that were extremely difficult for us to go through, I am happy to say that Peter and I are still friends to this day. He is now married to Melissa, a lovely woman whom I consider to be a friend. Peter and I have always remained a team in raising our sons, and that would become a crucial element to help us navigate all that we would go through with Zach.

Still, there I was not fitting in again; I was a single mom in my 40's with four little boys. I didn't have one friend at that time who was divorced, and it was a very lonely time for me, when I wasn't with my boys. I had been a stay at home mom for eight years and was grateful that I was able to do that, but it was time for me to get back to working. I began teacher training for pilates on the reformer, first in classical pilates, and later in Stott pilates. In 2008, my good friend Patty talked me into becoming a partner in a fairly new pilates studio in Orchard Park, called the Pilates Co-op. Peter was starting kindergarten, so it was perfect timing, and I was home every day by the time the boys were home from school. It was a booming business, and I had lovely clients, but I found myself still searching for "my thing," my life's purpose.

And so my spiritual journey began. I was still struggling with depression and began to go to a Hawaiian healer named Harry Jim who my sister recommended. Harry has a presence that is larger than life; he fills a room with his light. He is a gifted healer, and he helped me so much. He introduced me to breathing techniques, and I learned how we can shift our energy with our breath, and even heal trauma. I had also been practicing yoga for years, which helped me immensely. In yoga, we use our breath (or prana) in yoga poses to shift our energy. I loved the flow of vinyasa yoga because it felt like dancing to me. Yoga helped me to feel the "mind, body, spirit" connection that I had been searching for, and I knew I was on the right path.

I decided to become a yoga teacher, and did my yoga teacher training through the Downward Dog Yoga Centre in Toronto with Diane Bruni and Ron Reid. The first level was in Toronto for ten days, and then I completed the 200 RYT certification in Puerto Escondido, Mexico. This experience was life changing for me. Learning yoga from Diane and Ron was a gift; they are beautiful souls and incredible teachers. Diane has since crossed over and I am so grateful that I got to know her and learn from her. Participating in these yoga teacher trainings obviously helped me to learn how to teach, but beyond that, it helped me to heal. We were in a town in Mexico in the middle of nowhere, with no hotels or even street lights, immersed in yoga for seven hours a day with like-minded people. Every night, I was exhausted from the emotional releasing and healing. When I left that experience, I was starting to feel like my old self again … the girl who was joyful.

I left the pilates studio in 2010 and opened a yoga studio in Hamburg, New York called Lotus Yoga. I shared a space with my sister Kerry who is a massage therapist and gifted healer. Back then, yoga had not caught on yet in the southtowns of Buffalo as it had in other parts of the country. It definitely wasn't the trend that it is today. I know there were people who thought that I was crazy leaving a successful pilates business, but I had to follow my path. As Harry Jim always says, "What other people think of you is none of your business!" It's still one of my favorite sayings.

For the next few years, I read every spiritual book that I came upon. Some of the most impactful books for me were *Many Lives, Many Masters* by Brian Weiss, *The Untethered Soul* by Michael Singer, and *A New Earth* by Eckhart Tolle. The idea that we are all souls just having a life experience on earth helped me to see everything from a new perspective. The notion that there is only one God (whether you say God, or Allah, or "The Universe", etc), and that we all come from that divine energy, made sense to me. I studied the chakras and how they related to yoga poses and to our health. Above all, I believe that everything that I had gone through, and the tools that I had learned to help lift me out of depression, would later be crucial for me in managing everything I would go through with Zach.

PART 2

Zach's Story

"You wonderful boy, you brave, brave man."
- Harry Potter and the Deathly Hallows, J.K. Rowling

CHAPTER FOUR

Zach would tell me later on in his life that he had a happy childhood. He would thank me for that. His brothers were the biggest part of that. I have always told my boys that the greatest gift I've ever given them is each other. I always hoped that they would not only love each other, but like each other as well. That they certainly did.

They always had fun at home together, whether they were playing sports or watching tv shows on Disney channel or Nickelodeon, or watching their favorite movies. They loved *The Replacements*, *Remember the Titans*, all the *Star Wars* movies, and every *Harry Potter* movie.

Zach was obsessed with *Harry Potter* movies from the time he was 6. In fact, for his 7th birthday party, we took a pack of his friends (along with Christopher and Eric) to see the second *Harry Potter* movie in the theatre. It was probably completely inappropriate for Eric, but no way was he missing out! They became our family's favorite movies, and we all went together to the theatre to see each one as they came out. I cried at the end of the last movie, not just for the end of the *Harry Potter* era, but because it was the end of an era for us as well. The boys were getting older and would no longer want to see all their favorite movies with their mom and dad. Zach always reminded me of Harry Potter when he was a boy: kind, strong, quietly brave. Those qualities would become even more prevalent as he grew up.

There is no doubt that my boys' strongest bond was through sports. Their friend Ryan told me recently that he has never seen brothers so bonded by sports. They would watch endless hours of sports, discussing plays and players, and arguing over who was the best athlete. The endless argument of Kobe (Christopher's favorite) versus LeBron (Eric's favorite) always made Zach laugh.

They all played sports from the age of four through high school. While it may have been a foreign world for this ex-ballet dancer, I knew how good sports were for all of my sons. They were all high energy (even more so when they were all together!), and I believe the energy they exerted in sports helped them to be more focused in school and in life. Sports taught them discipline and the value of hard work. Most importantly, it taught them about teamwork and friendship. So many of their coaches throughout the years, including their dad, were exemplary men who taught them valuable life lessons.

They played all of the sports that Peter had played: baseball, basketball, and football. They also took swim lessons, golf lessons, and swim team at Wanakah, a local country club, when they were young. This was a foreign concept for me, as my family could not afford a country club when I was growing up, but I was fortunate to get to spend every day of summer with them while they did lessons and swim team. They loved it. My boys don't have any first cousins, but they were very close to their second cousins Angie, Delaney, Michael and Jonathan. Zach was especially close to them; they were all around his age, they grew up together, and they loved doing swim team and spending summers together. Zach would remain close to them throughout his entire life.

Wanakah is also where Zach found his love and talent for swimming. He was a natural at the butterfly, and it was beautiful to watch. He excelled at swimming and he won many races and medals over the years. I know that those summer days at Wanakah were happy times for Zach. He was very loved by his coaches and teammates.

There was no sport Zach loved more than football. It was one of the loves of his life. My boys all caught the football bug from their dad, who played right through college. When Zach wanted to start Little Loop Football at age 7, I cried. What if he got hurt? What if he got a concussion? I lost the argument. I was outvoted. Zach begged to play and Peter coached him, and all of our boys, for as long as they all played Little Loop.

Little Loop Football practice was five nights a week in August, to every mother's annoyance, but for Zach to have that bonding time with his dad every day was a blessing. By the time all of our boys were playing, we had four football games, back to back, every Saturday. It was complete insanity, but Zach loved every minute of it.

He excelled at football, and I believe that gave him a newfound confidence. The boy who used to nervously chew on his swim goggles during swim meets, was coming out of his shell. Football gave Zach the confidence that performing had given me. It also deepened his bond with his dad and his brothers even further. They all watched each other's games as well. For years, they have relived big games and funny stories together. For Zach, his Little Loop years were some of his happiest memories. He always said that Little Loop was when football was the most fun.

If I have given the impression that Zach was a saint, or any of my boys for that matter, let me dispel that myth right now. They were all mischievous, just like their dad had been. I clearly remember going to Zach's kindergarten parent/teacher conference. I couldn't wait to hear all the glowing compliments about my super smart, sweet, polite child. The teacher spent most of the session talking about how Zach and his friends were fooling around in the garden and knocked over the statue of the Blessed Mary. (This was a Catholic school after all.) I was devastated, as all moms are when they hear that their child isn't perfect. And so it began.

Next came ding-dong-ditching. This became an Olympic event in Peter's neighborhood; kids from all over Orchard Park came to ding-dong-ditch there, particularly since there was a grumpy man who would call the police on them. Clearly you live in a low crime town when the police respond to ding-dong-ditching complaints. The Liberatore boys typically got blamed for it since there were four of them and their dad lived right there, even though half the time that it happened they were at my house. To this day, if you get all of those boys together reminiscing about the ding-dong-ditching days, they are doubled over in laughter.

It was around that time that Zach and his friends starting getting in trouble in middle school. We were called in for a meeting to discuss intentional burping, ball throwing, and pencil tossing in school. Again, I probably overreacted since this was my oldest child. After raising four sons, I now know that most middle school aged boys are immature and obnoxious at times. Also, this particular private Catholic school at that time, had no idea how to handle 6th, 7th, and 8th grade boys. Still, I didn't like the idea of Zach being rude to teachers and this was a huge red flag for me.

While many people would say that that it's normal for a 7th grade boy to be acting up in school, a mom has instincts about her child, and I knew that this wasn't Zach. Something was going on with him. I wondered if it was the divorce. I had always suggested counseling for my boys, but they always declined, and we were always fortunate to have Francine as their "counselor." I suggested to Zach that it would probably be helpful for him to talk with a counselor, since it had been helping me. He agreed to it and began seeing someone who my counselor recommended.

She was a young, intelligent mom and Zach really liked her. My favorite part was that she suggested that Zach and I start writing to each other in a notebook. It was always easier for him to write about his feelings, and this was way before texting came about. He really opened up to me in that notebook; we actually used it on and off for many years, and I am writing this now in that very notebook.

She felt that Zach was very well adjusted to the divorce; he had a good relationship with his dad and lots of family time. She said that Zach's biggest issue was that he had severe anxiety. This was a shock to us. He had always been somewhat serious, and a worrier, but severe anxiety?? She said that he also had social anxiety, which explained why he would do things to get into trouble with his friends to make people laugh. It was easier to fit in that way.

He wrote in our notebook about his anxiety. He wrote that he worried about the future; he was worried about choosing a high school, worried about getting through high school, then choosing a college, and then going to college and being away from his family. He worried about growing up and finding a job. This was a lot of worry for a boy who was just starting 8th grade. Of course his dad and I told him that we would take it one step at a time, and that he would always have our help and support.

Because of the fact that we weren't happy with how his school was handling things, we switched him to the public middle school for 8th grade. By this time he had many friends at both schools, and he was happy to make the switch. His crew included his best friend Danny, Colin, Dillon, Sam, Bubba, and Joe. He seemed happy at his new school and decided to stop seeing his counselor.

It was the summer of 2010, and there was a lot of change on the horizon. It was the summer I was introduced to Keith, who seven years later would become my fiancé and move in with us. Yes, I am a slow mover. My friend Annmarie says that I am slow like a turtle. Keith was smart and handsome and funny but the truth is, my boys always came first and they were at an age where they still needed me all of the time, which left me with very little free time. Keith and I broke up several times over the years because of that, but he was there for most of all the football and basketball seasons, as well as much of what we went through with Zach.

It was also the summer that Zach prepared to start high school. He had a difficult time choosing which high school to go to. Coming from the private elementary school, most of the boys there were going to attend Canisius High School in the city of Buffalo, a private school, but Zach had many friends in Orchard Park and considered going to Orchard Park High School as well. He chose Canisius.

We will never know if that was the right decision for him. While CHS is a wonderful high school with some truly exemplary male teachers, many of whom inspired Zach, it was also a college prep school with more pressure on grades and college acceptance. I'm not saying the pressure came from the school itself, however at that time, many parents were placing great emphasis on SAT scores, GPA, and what college their child got into. I remember waiting to pick Zach up from freshman football practice and the parents behind me were discussing what GPA and SAT scores were required to get into Duke University. The thought crossed my mind that this type of atmosphere may not be ideal for a boy with high anxiety about the future, however he had made his choice.

Let me reiterate: Canisius is a top notch school, providing an excellent education, much support from the staff, and a true brotherhood. Zach's closest friends in life were his Canisius friends; Danny, Nolan, Troy, Sam B., Sam P., Chris, Adam, Connor, and Dillon. In retrospect, I just wonder if it added to his anxiety; yet another thing I've had to "let go" of.

The big excitement for all of us was that Zach was starting high school football. After seven years of Little Loop football, our family couldn't wait to go to high school games. Zach had always been a running back and cornerback because he was fast, but trying out for the Canisius team, he knew that there would be kids coming from all over Western New York and some would be faster than him, so he decided to go out for the quarterback position. Again, I thought, more pressure.

It's absolutely crazy how time flies when you have children. There is a saying, "When you have kids, the days are long, but the years fly by." No truer words. On the first day of high school, I drove Zach in. I can clearly recall looking over at him during the long drive, and he was sound asleep in his button down shirt and tie. When Zach was a toddler, he wouldn't nap in the crib anymore, only in the car. Every afternoon, I would take him for a drive so that he would sleep for a bit. For the rest of his life, he would instantly fall asleep in the car if the drive was longer than 15 minutes. I remember looking over at this boy who was becoming a man, thinking where did the time go? Of course I cried.

Initially his high school experience started out great. He made excellent grades, even with hours of homework every night, which he didn't even start until he got home from football practice late in the evening. He had an exciting football season as starting quarterback. It was so wonderful to see him step up as leader of the team. They had an undefeated season.

One of my proudest moments as a mom was at Zach's freshman football banquet. Zach was awarded most valuable player which I know he was very proud of, but more importantly, his coach described him as a leader with outstanding character. This was the Zach that I knew and after the past couple years of him misbehaving in school, it was such a relief to hear that he was maturing.

Sophomore year he was the starting QB again. It was another great season, in which they only lost one game. In the last game of the season, Zach threw the game winning touchdown at St. Francis High School. He was elated. He loved his team, and was always very hard on himself when he felt that he had "let the team down." Of course we always reminded him that it was just a game, and that since he was always giving 100%, there is no way he ever let the team down. Still, he always put that pressure on himself, so when they finished the season on such a high note, he was very proud, especially with his dad and all of his brothers there.

That same year he began dating Haley, a beautiful girl, inside and out. She was the younger sister of Bubba, one of his best friends. His life seemed good. I remember that Keith and I were sitting at one of Christopher's Canisius basketball games (he went to Canisius for two years and then decided to switch over to Orchard Park High School), and Zach and Haley walked in and sat in the front row. Keith noticed that literally every person who walked in, whether a student, teacher, or parent, broke into a huge smile when they saw Zach and shook his hand, or high-fived him. He always had that effect on people. Watching him that night, it looked like he had the perfect life, but that was far from the truth.

CHAPTER FIVE

In the spring of 2012, when Zach was 16 years old, I received a text from him:

I think I have OCD.

My brain tried to rationalize it. He had always had small signs of OCD. We thought that they were idiosyncrasies. When he was a small child, he couldn't stand for his clothes to be wet; I always had a spare set of clothes in the car in case he spilled something on himself. He always lined up his small toy animals just right. He never liked to eat when his dad's newspapers were strewn across the kitchen table. He never made a big deal about it, but I could tell that was the reason he didn't want to eat. When he was older, he never liked when the cap was off a water bottle or Gatorade bottle. The boys would mock him (as brothers do), "Ooooh look Zach, the cap is off." We would laugh.

These "quirks" were similar to my own, growing up. I've never been comfortable when there is clutter around me. Like Zach, I have never liked when my clothes or socks are wet. When I was dancing, I had to tie my pointe shoe ribbons a specific way so that I would have a good performance. When I got his text that day, my brain rationalized that Zach just had OCD tendencies like I did, and yet I felt the blood drain from my face because my instincts told me that something was very wrong.

Apparently, Zach had shared with Haley what some of his symptoms were, and they looked it up. He explained some of his symptoms to me as well, but did not disclose how bad it really was. He described his preoccupation with certain numbers, and how he had difficulty in school because his brain told him he could only use certain numbers in math. He also told me that when he was writing, the letters had to be formed perfectly, or he would have to start over and over. This would explain why his grades had started to drop. He described his brain's need for "symmetry." If his arm accidentally hit a wall, he felt that he had to hit the other arm as well. This need for symmetry also affected his driving; if he ran over a line on one side, his brain told him he had to run over the line on the other side.

He went back to seeing his mental health counselor, and she also suggested that we consult our physician about starting him on medication for anxiety. We resisted and had a bad feeling about it, but our son was suffering and wanted relief so we gave in. Our pediatrician started him on a low dose of Zoloft. In the meantime, I tried other healing modalities with him, some of the things that had always helped me. I took him to see Harry Jim, my Hawaiian healer. I took him for accupuncture. He even tried yoga with me.

He seemed to be doing okay, or at least that's what he wanted us to think, until a few months later when he admitted that none of this was helping at all. He admitted that he hadn't fully disclosed all of his symptoms to his counselor, or told her how bad things really were. He told us that his life was a living hell. Of course as his mom, I already knew that he wasn't doing well. He kept insisting up to that point that he was okay because he didn't want to worry or scare us. Now we were worried, and we were scared.

Herein lies the truth of having a child with mental illness; you have no idea where to go or who to turn to for help. If your child has a broken arm, you go to the hospital. If your child has cancer, you find the best cancer institute. Eleven years ago in Buffalo, it was impossible to know what to do for our child who had severe obsessive-compulsive disorder. We didn't know ANYONE who had any experience with it. There was no OCD "clinic" that we knew of in Western New York. We consulted psychiatrists and psychologists who treated OCD and for anyone we found, there was at least a month waitlist. This would not do. He needed immediate help.

We researched OCD online of course. There is no definitive cause. It can possibly be a brain abnormality, and /or hereditary. During that time, I realized that both of our families had a history of OCD; hoarding is a form of OCD. Severe OCD is usually treated with a combination of medication and therapy, often Cognitive Behavioral Therapy (CBT) and Exposure and Response Prevention (ERP). All of this sounded vaguely familiar from my four years in psychology at college, but I could never have known back then that I would be experiencing this firsthand with my own son.

A friend of mine referred us to a psychiatric nurse practitioner who could help with the medication while we waited the month for the appointment with the psychologist. The appointment with the PNP was still a two week wait and I felt like the worst mother in the world, seeing my son in pain and telling him to wait a couple of weeks for help. We counted the days down. Zach spent most of his time at my house, even when his brothers were at their dad's house. It was his safe place and he didn't want to be around people. He spent all of his time in his room when he wasn't at school.

Finally the day came for the PNP appointment. Peter and I told Zach that in order for this woman to be able to help him, he had to be completely honest with her. He had to tell her everything. He wrote down three pages of obsessions and compulsions to show her and he let us read them. We were speechless. We just looked at each other, crushed that our boy lived like this. Peter said to me, "How does he get through a day?" How could we not have known? Three pages of obsessive thoughts and compulsions that had taken over his life. He had difficulty getting through school days, it affected his driving, and he couldn't even spend time with his friends or girlfriend anymore.

I took Zach to the appointment and he went in with the PNP first, along with his list of obsessions and compulsions. It was a long time before she called me in. She told me that Zach had very severe OCD and that only high doses of medications were effective in treating it, so the low does of Zoloft that he had been on wasn't helping at all. She would increase his dose, however this had to be done slowly and could take 4-6 weeks before it actually helped. (WHAT?!) She strongly advised that he keep the upcoming appointment with the psychologist, even though he didn't specialize in OCD, because meds plus therapy usually had the best outcome.

Then she dropped the bomb. She quietly and slowly told me that Zach had serious thoughts of taking his own life. I froze and just stared at her. There was complete silence. This could not be true. I turned to look at Zach beside me. His head was hanging down and he slowly looked up into my eyes. In those beautiful eyes I saw sadness, fear, regret, and guilt. It was true then. My beautiful boy wanted to end his life. He never told us of course. He never wanted to be a burden, or to cause us pain. He was ashamed that he had these thoughts. My heart hurt with the knowledge that he had been carrying this alone, so typical of Zach.

She told Zach that in the interim of waiting for the meds to kick in, if he needed immediate help, he should call the suicide hotline. I had to go home and tell Peter that our boy's life was such a living hell, he didn't want to live anymore. I don't even remember what we told Christopher, Eric and Peter. I know that we told them about the severe OCD, but didn't disclose the whole truth. It was too much, too scary. They certainly knew that their big brother had not been well for a long time and they were scared, but they tried not to show it.

It was now Christmas season 2012. We celebrated Zach's 17th birthday. We were in a haze of fear and watched him day and night for signs of him getting worse. I constantly asked him if he was okay. The holidays were a blur, as we tried to make it fun for the other boys.

One day in early January, Zach said that he was "not good." (For the next 8 years, whenever Zach said he was "not good," we knew how bad that really was.) He looked scared. We suggested he call the suicide hotline as the PNP had recommended and he did. He spoke at length with someone who finally ascertained that he needed immediate help and she told him to go to Erie County Medical Center (ECMC).

It was evening, so I took Zach alone and Peter stayed with the boys. They were 14,12, and 10, but it was too frightening of a situation to leave them home alone. There are many things in my life that I cannot recall, but I remember every moment of that night as if it happened yesterday. We went to the ER at ECMC and we were sent to the Children's Psychiatric Emergency Room where Zach was evaluated.

The attending psychiatrist saw him alone first and then they brought me in. He wanted to admit Zach to the Child's Psychiatric Inpatient Unit because he had been having suicidal thoughts while driving and feared that he would drive himself right into a tree and kill himself.

He also put Zach on Klonopin in addition to the Zoloft he was already taking. My blood ran cold when he talked about Klonopin. My intuition told me it wasn't good. Klonopin is a benzodiazepine ("benzo") and he was giving it to Zach to help with his extreme state of anxiety and panic attacks. Side effects for Klonopin can include dependency and addiction to the drug. The psychiatrist was only trying to help Zach so I'm not blaming him in any way, but after that, Zach became dependent on Klonopin for the rest of his life.

We waited in the tiny waiting room for hours for him to be admitted. It was 3 am by the time we went up to the Child's Psychiatric Unit. The nurse took his shoes and the drawstring from his sweatpants, since shoelaces and drawstrings can potentially be used by a patient to hang himself. It was surreal. It was terrifying. After he was admitted, I was told that I had to leave him at the doors to the unit and that I wasn't allowed to go any further. We stood at the big doors that would barricade him in and just stared at each other. I could hear in the background one of the nurses saying to another, "They're so cute." I hugged him tight and said the only thing that I could think of, "Everything will be okay. I love you so much."

"Love you too. Bye mom," he said.

I prayed, "God, please heal my Zach."

As they bolted the big doors behind me, I could still see him watching me leave, just like he did when he was in pre school. I mustered the biggest smile I could and waved confidently at him and then I ran. I ran through the dark, silent hospital because I couldn't breathe. I was terrified. How long would they keep him there? We both had to sign paperwork stating that it was up to the doctors to determine when he could leave. I now knew what anxiety felt like, as if my insides were shaking. And so, our nightmare began.

On the long drive home, I was still shaking, but something incredible happened. Zach had always been a huge music lover. He loved all kinds of music, many different genres. He loved the Beatles and Bob Marley. He was into Drake and Eminem before I ever heard of them. Johnny Cash was one of his favorites and he watched the movie *Walk the Line* many times. At that time, one of his favorite songs was *Home* by Phillip Phillips. Phillips had won *American Idol* and he was Zach's favorite from the very beginning of the show. Whenever I heard *Home* it always reminded me of Zach. On that night, as I was crying all the way home, I heard *Home* on the radio no less than five times. It would end, I would change the channel, and it would be playing on another channel. There is no doubt in my mind that my angels and guides were giving me a clear sign. Zach would be okay.

For the next two weeks our life was put on hold as Peter and I took turns going up to the hospital to see Zach. I canceled all of my yoga classes. I spent every moment worrying about him. I thought that's what I was supposed to do. We were allowed to visit at lunch and dinner and we would bring his favorite take out foods to cheer him up. Zach and I would play scrabble for the entire visit.

His high school was back in session and they were very supportive of his absence. I was surprised to hear from his school counselor that Zach was not the first Canisius student to have spent time at the ECMC Children's Psychiatric Unit. Father Betti, the resident priest at CHS at that time, whom all the boys loved, was the first to ask if he could visit Zach.

One of the hardest aspects of all of this for our family, was the complete unknown. We didn't know of a single child who had gone to a psych unit because of suicidal thoughts. We didn't know anyone who struggled with severe OCD or high anxiety or any mental illness the way that Zach did. It was really difficult trying to explain to close friends and family and beyond that, we didn't really tell other people. There was also a stigma attached to mental illness and as his parents, we tried to protect him from that.

It would have been comforting to have had someone to talk to who understood what we were going through. There were probably people we knew who had gone through similar situations, but if there were, we had never heard about it. In the past decade since Zach was at ECMC, I know of at least 25 kids in my community alone who have struggled with mental illness and addiction. I don't know if there are more kids now who have anxiety disorders and depression, or if it is just talked about more openly now.

At the end of two weeks, Zach was released and we met with the head psychiatrist to formulate a plan for his return to "normal" life. We were incredibly fortunate to have her link Zach to a psychologist who specialized in OCD at the Children's Psychiatric Clinic of Oishei Children's Hospital. I was hopeful, but I could see the fear in Zach's eyes. He was clearly afraid that leaving this safe environment would lead him right back to where he had been before, and his OCD was not any better.

When Zach came home, we all watched him with trepidation. We tried to keep it positive with the boys but they were obviously worried about their big brother. There is a moment I remember very clearly when Zach was having a really bad day soon after he arrived home. He was in the bathroom for hours with many of his OCD compulsions and he came down wearing my white bathrobe. He sat at the dining room table, hunched over and crying uncontrollably. Christopher was bouncing a ball in the foyer behind him. (Please no judgement on the ball bouncing in the house.) I watched Christopher bouncing as if he was on a basketball court, moving back and forth and all around, never taking his eyes off of Zach and not

saying a word. My heart broke for both of them; my son who lived with so much pain, and my son who was in pain worrying about his big brother.

I took Christopher aside and told him that we were getting Zach the help he needed and that he was going to be okay. I think that is the only time that I broke a promise to one of my sons.

CHAPTER SIX

For the next 8 1/2 years, this would be our new "normal." Life was insanely busy with our four sons in school and sports, but for our family, time would stand still when Zach was doing really badly. When he was doing better, I was good. When he was not good, I was not good. We all watched him constantly, searching for signs that he was at a low point. We all became very in tune to how he was, even though Zach usually tried to hide his pain. In our writing to each other over the years, Zach often told me that he never wanted to be a burden to his family. He didn't want all the family's energy and attention to be directed at him, but that's just how it was.

In February of 2013, he began going to his new psychologist at the Children's Psychiatric Clinic. Zach liked him a lot and said that he helped him. He would be his patient for the next five years. Because it was a children's clinic, I was part of Zach's appointments for the better part of five years. He would have time alone with the psychologist and then I would come in at the end to discuss how the session went. The psychologist explained that there would always be peaks and valleys for Zach. We, his family, came to know all the signs of his valleys.

It is with a heavy heart that I say that Zach's "peaks" were never that high. From the time he was 16 until the day he died, he was never "good." Some days weren't as bad as others; some days he managed his OCD. I don't think anyone knew Zach as well as I did. The bond we always shared enabled me to instinctively know when he was suffering, even if he tried to hide it. There is nothing harder as a parent than watching your child suffer and not be able to help him. We tried to get him the help he needed, and he tried to get better, but his pain was something that I carried for many years. I know that his dad did too.

In the spring of Zach's junior year, he appeared to be doing somewhat better than he had been. His new psychologist helped him to manage his OCD symptoms and the new medications helped slightly. He helped his dad coach Peter's Little League Baseball games, which Peter loved. He went to a prom with his friends. Things were looking up, until Peter and I were called in to a meeting at school with Zach, the dean of students, and the head coach of the varsity football team. Zach had gotten into trouble for drinking with another student in Orchard Park and CHS had heard about it. We also knew that Zach had been smoking marijuana. He was reprimanded at school and we grounded him for both incidences, but clearly he was starting to "self medicate." One more thing for us to watch for and worry about.

The main reason they wanted to talk with us however, was to see how Zach was doing mentally. They had a big question to ask him. They wanted him to be the starting quarterback for the varsity football team for the upcoming season, Zach's senior year. The word "NO!" immediately came out of my mouth. All eyes were on this team. They had been undefeated in Western New York for two years. This was way too much pressure on a kid who just got out of the psychiatric ward at ECMC three months earlier.

Of course Zach immediately said yes and the decision was his to make. Once they were old enough, we have never tried to coerce our sons into doing what we want them to do. We let them choose what high school they wanted to go to and what college they wanted to go to (within reason financially). I always suggested music lessons, piano lessons, instruments, and musical theatre (wishful thinking!), but always let them choose what extracurricular activity they wanted to do. They all obviously chose football, basketball, and baseball. I have always believed that as parents, we are given these little humans to nurture, but they are actually fully grown souls and should be allowed to choose their own path, not what we think their path should be. Peter and I both have always tried to support our boys in whatever they chose.

Zach wanted to be the quarterback of this team. The most interesting thing about football for Zach was that when he was playing, it was the only time that he did not have OCD symptoms. For whatever reason, he was so focused on the plays, that his mind could be quiet and not have the OCD thoughts. It was almost meditative for him, just as yoga was for me. Unfortunately he never found anything else that could quiet his mind like that, which is why he would turn to alcohol and painkillers.

The summer of 2013 was incredibly busy for Zach. He always seemed to be better when he was busy and he seemed to be doing okay. He had a job at Towne Auto washing cars, he had football practice almost every day, and he also had to complete senior community service hours for CHS, since he wouldn't have time once football season began.

There was a tournament held every year at St. John Fisher College in Rochester which preceded the start of fall football. Canisius won the tournament that summer with Zach as the starting quarterback. Unfortunately for Zach, right after that CHS brought in a QB from Canada who would apparently be competing with Zach for the starting QB position. As the season opener approached, there was still no word as to who would be the starting QB. This was obviously a blow to Zach. In addition to that, Canisius was featured not only on the front page of the sports section of the Buffalo News, but also on the front page of the paper! They had been undefeated for two years and were ranked #1 in the state of New York. The pressure was on.

As Zach's senior football season began, it felt like Peter and I were holding our breath with trepidation. As excited as we were, we watched

Zach closely. He considered quitting the team because of the indecision about who the quarterback would be. We told him that it was obviously his choice, but he would probably always regret missing his senior year of football, not to mention letting down his teammates that he had come to love. He decided to stay with it and I know that he never regretted that decision.

Peter and I were incredibly proud of Zach that football season, for many reasons. Even though he was struggling with his constant OCD plus anxiety over the intense pressure, he dug down deep and he persevered. He and Jake, the other QB, alternated games, drives, and sometimes even plays, but they became friends and led their team to an almost perfect season.

They lost a big game against Aquinas High School in Rochester, a highly competitive team. The next day, there was a huge picture of Zach in the Buffalo News, literally upside down in the air as he was being tackled. What we remember most about that game was Zach's relentless strength and courage. He never gave up, and he played with such heart until the bitter end.

Another big game was against Cardinal Mooney High School in Ohio. Zach injured his hand in that game but continued to play. The coaches were afraid his hand was broken, so they asked us to drive him back to Buffalo immediately after the game for X-rays, rather than have him take the bus back with the team.

As we were waiting for Zach to get dressed, my son Peter and I ran into Tyrone Wheatley, an NFL coach and former NFL player whose son TJ was one of Zach's teammates. (TJ now plays in the NFL and Zach was SO proud of him and honored to have been his teammate.) Tyrone told Peter and me that Zach was one of the toughest kids he had ever seen, and that if he could take Zach's "heart" and put it in every player's body, they would be the best team in the country. Peter and I just looked at each other in amazement, totally speechless. Did nobody else hear that??!! I wish I could have videotaped it for Zach to see! Truth be told, when I was trying to recall exactly what Tyrone had said, my son Peter remembered every word.

The six of us squeezed into Peter's truck for the four hour drive back to

Buffalo to get Zach's hand X-rayed. When I told Zach what Tyrone Wheatley had said, he was on cloud nine. I don't think I have ever seen Zach so proud of himself as he was at that moment. He smiled through the entire long drive. It is a shining example of how someone's kind words can impact a person.

Another really exciting game was the rivalry game against St. Joe's Collegiate of Buffalo. At that time, it was ranked to be one of the top rivalries in the country. Thousands of people came to these games and it was quite exciting. Zach's team won that day. My dad was at that game and one of my favorite photos of all time is a picture of Zach and him, my dad beaming with pride. It was incredible to see Zach confidently walk across the field with his beautiful smile, and nobody knew what he was really going through.

In Western New York, all of the high school football championships are played at the Buffalo Bills stadium in Orchard Park. As you can imagine, this is a dream come true for young football players. All three of my sons who played varsity football (Eric dropped football to focus on basketball) got to play at the championship game at the Bills stadium. How lucky were they!

Zach's team won the Monsignor Martin Championship that year. He played a great game. I have photos of him throwing a pass on the Bills emblem on the field. After the game, I took a photo of Zach with his brothers. It was by far, one of the happiest moments of his life. I don't think I have ever seen him happier. It was a memory that I know he always cherished.

It wasn't just about winning. I recently found a manuscript about his life that Zach had started writing years ago. In it he wrote: *That team made me a better man, and helped me understand the feeling of a true brotherhood, aside from actual blood relation.*

He loved that team, especially Dillon, Colin, Josh, Brad, Connor, Deanthony, Keon, Pat, and Ryan. He also loved his coaches. I ran into his head coach when Zach had gotten into trouble at school for some immature behavior and he said to me, "Zach is a good soul." Yes. He understood Zach and I will always be grateful to him and the other coaches and his team-mates for giving him that time in his life. He was a leader and a warrior during that football season, and perhaps that is what propelled him to be a leader and a warrior later in his life.

Unfortunately, as soon as football season was over, Zach mentally started going downhill again. His OCD escalated again and he probably didn't tell us until he could barely function. In mid holiday season, he told us that he needed help. He needed to go to inpatient immediately to keep himself safe because he was having suicidal thoughts again. It had been suggested to us that if he needed inpatient help again, Brylin Hospital in Buffalo was another option along with ECMC where he had gone the previous year. Zach called Brylin, did the interview, and they had a bed available for him.

So on a cold winter night, I left Zach at yet another inpatient treatment facility. Brylin brought up painful memories for me as my dad had done treatment there for alcoholism twice when I was in high school. Now it was strictly for mental illness. We did the same intake procedure that we would become painfully familiar with over the years. He did more evaluations and paperwork before he had to hand over his shoelaces and then was taken upstairs. I prayed, "God, please heal my Zach."

Brylin is a short term facility; typically a patient is kept on average of five days, just to keep them safe. I would soon become uncomfortably familiar with the routine of checking him in and riding the elevator upstairs for visiting hours. In the next six years, Zach would check himself into Brylin four more times. It became a "safe" place for him when he was having suicidal thoughts. Peter and I would juggle the boys' schedules while alternating going up to visit him. Having a child who has suicidal thoughts, there is an element of relief in knowing that they are locked up and safe at an inpatient facility, but at the same time, there is just fear. Always fear.

He came home in time to celebrate his 18th birthday and Christmas. His last few months of high school were a roller coaster of emotions for all of us. Zach had received his college acceptance letters and he was adamant that he wanted to attend Duquesne University in Pittsburgh for business.

Of course we questioned the notion of Zach going to college 3 1/2 hours away, given his severe struggles. His psychologist strongly recommended that Zach make his own decision and that we should support him.

He had always considered playing college football at the D3 level, but when the time came, he didn't pursue it and did not apply to any schools where he would be able to play. Duquesne was D1 and out of his league. I am sure that his severe OCD, anxiety, and depression played into his decision, but he would admit years later that he wished he had played football in college. As his parents, it broke our hearts that the option was taken away from him because of the state of his mental health.

In March, I took him to the accepted business students orientation at Duquesne. We toured the campus, we walked around the city of Pittsburgh, and I took photos of him at his new school. It should have been exciting, but I knew that we were both nervous.

I have always been a sentimental crybaby mama bear when it comes to my boys growing up and all the "firsts" and "lasts": first day of kindergarten, last "first day of school," Senior Night for football and basketball, last prom, high school graduation, college graduation. People told me that I wouldn't cry when my youngest child went to kindergarten or graduated high school, but I cried just as hard when Peter went to kindergarten as I did when Zach went. It all just goes so fast and while I was always grateful that they were moving forward with their lives as they should, part of me always laments the days that are no more.

At Canisius High School they have a beautiful tradition for moms. Every spring there is a Mother/Son Dance, fondly referred to as the "Mom Prom." The last "Mom Prom" brought me to tears of course. The seniors danced with their moms to *I Hope You Dance* by Lee Ann Womack. There couldn't have been a more perfect song for us. All I hoped for my beautiful son was for him to "dance"; to be happy and at peace and to live his life. My friend Stephanie took a picture of us while we were dancing. I treasure it. It is the only photo I will ever have of us dancing together.

Zach was up and down during those final months before graduation.

His OCD was intense and severe and it was affecting his grades. We worried that he wouldn't even be able to graduate, which was crazy since every psychologist and psychiatrist he ever went to, deemed him highly intelligent.

Graduation day came and it was one of the happiest days of my life. It was a happy day for all of us, especially Zach. Peter and I literally high-fived each other when Zach crossed that stage to receive his diploma. It hadn't been easy to get to this point. We took all the photos afterward with our families and Zach's friends. We went to Hutch's for dinner, which is a restaurant in Buffalo that has always been my favorite, as well as Zach's favorite. It was one of those days that will forever be etched in my mind as the happiest of memories.

CHAPTER SEVEN

In THE SUMMER OF 2014, we knew that Zach was not doing well but as usual, had no idea how to help him. He said he was okay, but I knew better. It was his first summer in ten years without football and I knew that it hit him hard. It also left him with a lot of free time, which I knew from his psychology appointments was always difficult for him. He worked for his dad doing landscaping, but he had too much time on his hands to do nothing but worry about going away to college and how he would navigate that with his OCD compulsions.

He would be roommates with his good friend Troy from Canisius, so we were hopeful that would help. Zach and I went to student orientation with Troy and his mom, but I saw the worry in Zach's eyes. We continued to tell him that he did not have to go away to college. There are plenty of great colleges in WNY and he could live at home for awhile, or at least dorm close to home. He held firm in wanting to go to Duquesne.

He had his last appointment with his psychologist in Buffalo a week before he had to leave for Pittsburgh. They brought me in at the end of the appointment as usual to go over the plan moving forward, but on that day another bomb dropped. Nothing prepared me for what the psychologist would tell me. Zach had bulimia, and it was pretty severe. Bulimia? My son had bulimia? My son the football player had an eating disorder? I sat there completely speechless, trying to process it all.

According to the National Eating Disorders Association website, "Bulimia Nervosa is a serious, life-threatening eating disorder characterized by a cycle of binging and compensating behaviors such as self-induced vomiting designed to undo or compensate for the effects of binge eating."

I personally was all too familiar with eating disorders. I was a ballet dancer in New York City in the 80's and unfortunately the uber thin dancer was what was hired back then. I wouldn't say that I ever had a diagnosed eating disorder, but I definitely had bouts of starving myself during performance season. When I was dancing with Buffalo Ballet Theatre in high school, I would sometimes go days living on 300-400 calories a day, while dancing for four hours a day. My weight would get down very low, but after performance season, I would go back to my "normal" weight. This love/hate relationship with food lasted for many years, until I was pregnant with Zach. When I knew that I was feeding him too, I began to concern myself with healthy foods, rather than just counting calories.

I was surrounded by girls with eating disorders in my teens and 20's. It made me so sad to see so many beautiful and talented girls starving themselves to be thinner, in order to fit someone else's mold of what they should be. I wrote several papers about eating disorders in high school and in college. In fact, my intention after college was to go into counseling for eating disorders and although it didn't happen back then, I had LITERALLY just started graduate school at Canisius College in Buffalo for mental health counseling, and I had just written yet another paper on eating disorders.

So how could I have missed the fact that my own son had an eating disorder? He was definitely thinner, smaller, but we attributed that to the fact that he didn't play football anymore. He did spend a lot of time in the bathroom, but he had always done that with his OCD compulsions. I was overwhelmed with guilt that I had missed the signs. I had never even heard of a boy with an eating disorder. (However, since then many males in sports have opened up about their eating disorder.) I could tell that Zach was not only embarrassed to admit he had bulimia, but he also felt guilty to be dumping another problem on us. I saw it all in his eyes.

First and foremost, we had to discuss the fact that Zach was scheduled to move into his dorm at Duquesne in a week. His psychologist said that they had discussed it at length and that Zach felt that he had to at least try, or he would always regret it. However, his psychologist was adamant; if Zach got there and wanted to come home, then we were to bring him home. This was not a kid who we should force to "stick it out" for a semester if he didn't want to be there. He had been in a psych ward 18 months ago, had severe OCD, and severe bulimia.

As the days counted down for him to leave, I was secretly terrified but tried not to show it. Zach was clearly nervous. He didn't pack a thing. I bought all of his dorm stuff for him, and finally forced him to pack with me the day before we left. Peter and Petes and I drove Zach to Duquesne. We moved him into his dorm room with Troy. I went with him to the counseling center, which I had called ahead to alert them of Zach's situation. We took him out for dinner and walked around Pittsburgh and his campus, which was all so exciting for most students, but when Peter and I saw the communal bathroom for the dorm, we just looked at each other sadly. How would this work for Zach who would now have no privacy?

I held back the tears when I hugged him goodbye, and then cried for half the drive home. I know that most moms are emotional when their child goes off to college, but this was different. He wasn't happy and excited. His OCD was always a weight that held him down. For Peter and me, there was ALWAYS a fear that he would get to a point so low that he would take his life. The one constant that never wavered over the years is that Zach's safe place was home with his family. Every psychologist, every psychiatrist, every counselor he ever had, supported that. We were always his support system, especially his brothers. With him now being so far from home, I was scared.

The first few phone calls from him made us nervous. He was already struggling and we tried to be encouraging, but by day six, he wanted to come home. We did what his psychologist suggested and Peter went to bring him home. They pulled into my driveway and Zach was barely out of the car when Petes came flying out of the house and practically tackled Zach, the two of them grinning ear to ear. Petes was almost 12 at the time and he adored Zach. They were very close and at that moment I was positive we did the right thing in bringing him home.

Zach continued to get worse after that. We told him he had to enroll at SUNY Erie, the local community college until he figured out his next move. For all of the years after that, we always required Zach to either work full time, or go to college and work part time, even if he wasn't doing well. The doctors and counselors always said that it was essential to have structure and a schedule. He started at ECC, but whenever he wasn't there or at work, he was laying on the floor at my house. He became extremely depressed. I had heard of a counselor who specialized in eating disorders, so Zach began seeing her. After a few appointments, she told me that she had never had a client that she felt she couldn't help, until Zach. She said that most of her clients had some sort of trauma, often abuse, that was the root cause but Zach did not have this. His bulimia continued to worsen and his depression scared me to the point that I felt I had to leave the graduate program at Canisius, and to close my yoga studio and teach classes at home so that I could keep an eye on Zach. I moved my two pilates reformers into my small living room that nobody used and took pilates and yoga clients at home. It became our new normal.

Then when it seemed like things couldn't get much worse, tragedy struck. I was teaching a yoga class one morning at my house and when I turned my phone back on, there were frantic messages from Zach. Nolan Burch, one of his best friends, was in the hospital in West Virginia after a tragic hazing incident. Zach said that he didn't think Nolan was going to make it and he was already in his car on the way to West Virginia. Nolan's parents, Kim and TJ were already there and had called Zach. I called Zach and begged him to come back and let me drive with him, but he was already in Pennsylvania.

Nolan was a freshman at WVU and had been given a bottle of alcohol that he was required to drink at a fraternity hazing. He was discovered unconscious, but was not immediately taken to the hospital. The most heartbreaking thing was that Nolan's life could have been saved if 911 had been called sooner. His parents kept him on life support so that his organs could be donated.

Zach and a few of his friends were at the hospital with the Burch's and their daughter Alex, where they were able to say goodbye to their friend. Nolan had just had his 18th birthday. I didn't know Kim very well back then, but I just remember that I couldn't eat or sleep thinking about her losing her beautiful son. It was unthinkable. I didn't know how she could even get out of bed each morning. How could she even continue living? I had no idea of course that this was foreshadowing of what would happen to me six years later.

Zach was asked to be a pall bearer at Nolan's funeral. I took him to a men's store in town and bought him his first suit. It needed to be altered. I stood there watching him getting his first suit altered to wear to his friend's funeral. It felt so wrong. I was sick to my stomach and worried about Zach.

We were supposed to pick up the suit the next day, which was the day of the wake. Instead, we were hit with a monumental snowstorm, which would later be named "Snowvember." We would not be able to get the suit. Everything was shut down. Five feet of snow had fallen south of Buffalo where we lived. There was literally a wall of snow over Lake Erie and everywhere north of the wall barely got any snow. There was a driving ban in Orchard Park and some people were snowed in their homes. Regardless of the driving ban, I knew I had to get Zach to Nolan's services. He absolutely had to be there with his friends. Peter was out plowing his properties for 24 hours straight, so we left the boys snowed in at his house.

We got in the car and started driving through back roads to get to the Northtowns because the thruway was closed. The only cars on the road were police cars and plow trucks. I prayed we didn't spin off the road. I prayed we didn't get pulled over for being out on the road. By some miracle, we made it through to the area that was untouched by the storm and made it to the wake.

Kim and TJ were pillars of strength. I just remember watching Zach so closely, looking for signs of a breakdown. I was so grateful that he could be there with his friends and with Nolan's family. It would have been devastating for him if we wouldn't have been able to be there. He and his friends reminisced about Nolan and shared memories.

There was so much love and support for the Burch family. Nolan was very beloved at Canisius High School and in Amherst where he lived. He was truly a special soul. I asked my son Christopher what he remembered most about Nolan. He said, "Nolan had this crazy giggle when he was laughing, that made you laugh. He was always smiling. He was always cracking up all the boys." I also asked Zach's best friend Danny what he remembered most about his friend Nolan. He said, "His laugh was the absolute best in the world. He made friends with everybody wherever he went. He loved chewing tobacco with Z. He loved freestyle rapping at the end of the night. He loved torturing Alex (his sister) and his parents."

The funeral was on a freezing cold snowy morning. Zach and Danny and their crew were the pall bearers for their friend. It was tragic. It hurt too much to look at them. I didn't know how Kim and TJ were still standing. My heart broke for them. No parent should have to bury their child.

Not surprisingly, Zach sunk even deeper into depression after that. He had three framed photos on his dresser; a photo with his brothers after the championship game at the Bills stadium, a photo of Zach and his dad and me at football senior day, and a photo of Nolan and Danny and Zach that I took of them leaving for junior prom. Zach would just sit and stare at that photo. It was impossible to believe that Nolan was gone. All of Nolan's friends were devastated, but Zach was at rock bottom before Nolan died, so we were terrified of how he would handle it. The truth is, Zach never got over losing Nolan.

It was now holiday season 2014 and Zach barely left the house. His OCD was terrible as always, he was severely depressed, and he was losing weight by the week. Ever since Zach was a baby, we had a yearly Christmas tradition of making cut out cookies with my sister Kerry. She always took a picture of the boys with the inevitable frosting mess and finished cookies. (Some years the challenge was to make the ugliest cookies.) When I look back at the photo from that year, Zach was so thin, he didn't even look like himself.

He had been seeing both his psychologist for OCD and counselor for the eating disorder, plus a nutritionist, but he was clearly getting worse instead of better. It was suggested to us that an intensive inpatient eating disorder treatment facility may be what he needed. There was a facility in Rochester, but it was for females only. That was a common theme as we started to broaden our search. Not only that, he was 18 so he could only do an adult program which was even more difficult to find for a male. We were referred to a treatment center in Thousand Oaks, California called La Ventana.

La Ventana offered treatment for both males and females and they had a bed available. Zach did the intake and was accepted to their program. He could go immediately. We pressed him a little. Was he sure this was what he wanted to do? It was a 30 day inpatient, then PHP (Partial Hospitalization Program), and then IOP (Intensive Outpatient Program) which could be up to three months total, across the country from his family.

He was adamant that he wanted to go. He desperately wanted to get better. The combination of OCD and bulimia had made him a prisoner in his own home. As we celebrated his 19th birthday, we just wanted our boy to have a normal life with school and friends, and we worried about what he was doing to his body, his heart, and other organs.

I had researched bulimia at length. I spoke with the therapists there several times before he left, to make sure the OCD would be treated as well. They said that they often work with co-occurring disorders such as OCD and depression, which are common for those who struggle with an eating disorder, so that was hopeful for us. One of the therapists also asked me what his substance abuse problem was. I said that he didn't have a substance abuse problem. He used to drink on weekends with friends and he used to smoke marijuana, but hadn't done either of those in many months. She said that roughly 50% of individuals with an eating disorder (ED) has a problem with alcohol or drugs. I felt a chill go through my body. More foreshadowing. I could not, at that time, wrap my head around any more problems.

CHAPTER EIGHT

In January of 2015, Zach and I flew to California. He was quiet and nervous for the entire trip. I was too. I rented a car and drove in the dark through the hills to Thousand Oaks. He couldn't be admitted until morning, so we stayed at a hotel and headed out first thing in the morning. It was a beautiful area. Zach looked hopeful about that, especially since it was cold and gray in Buffalo at the time. We were both warm weather people and we both always preferred summer to winter in Buffalo.

When we arrived at the La Ventana office, we did the check in procedure. Zach had to have a full physical in Buffalo before he came, as well as the extensive mental health intake over the phone, so there wasn't much to do. I was only there for about an hour. It seemed crazy that I was leaving him there for treatment with complete strangers for the next 6-8 weeks. He walked me to my car to say goodbye before they would take him to the house where he would be living. I asked him if he was sure about this and he said yes. We hugged goodbye. I said, "Everything will be okay. I love you."

"Bye mom. Love you too."

I tried not to panic as I drove away. I prayed, "God, please heal my Zach." I had an entire day to kill since my flight wasn't until morning, so

I stopped at a mall. I wanted to get something that would remind me of Zach. I stopped at a store and saw an elephant bracelet in the case. I bought it to remind myself that Zach would be okay.

I stopped for an early dinner and was eating by myself when the call came from Zach. He was crying so hard, I could barely understand him. "Mom, please you have to come back and get me. I can't stay here. The food is awful and there is a lock on the bathroom door to keep us from using it, and I can't do this."

I tried to reason with him. I told him that it wouldn't be easy, but I knew he could do this. He had said that he wanted to get better. He had to give it a try and give it some time. He wasn't allowed to have his cell phone so he was using his limited time on the house phone and had to hang up. I didn't know what to do. I was about to drive back and get him, but I called Peter and texted my sister. Peter said, "You have to leave him there. He needs this. He wasn't getting any better in Buffalo." I knew that he was right. He needed intense inpatient treatment.

Then my sister Kerry texted me back, reminding me of something a spiritual teacher had said to me months ago, "You can throw a rope down to Zach, but he is the one who has to grab it and climb up the rope." Yes, she was right. That was true. I took what Peter and Kerry said as a sign and I left Zach there. I got on a five hour flight the next morning and I cried most of the way home. I believed that I was doing the best thing that I could for Zach, but I still felt guilty. I had spent 19 years trying to be the best mother my boys could have, and now I felt like a horrible mother.

For the next ten days, every time Zach had phone time, he called either Peter or me, begging us to let him come home. I had a constant stomach ache and dreaded his calls. We continuously reminded him that he needed this level of care and to give it time. Then it felt like a miracle happened. He called me and said he wanted to stay. He knew that it wouldn't be easy, but he liked the people there and he wanted to get better. He even apologized for giving us such a hard time. It was a huge turning point.

He kept saying that he only wanted to do the 30 day inpatient program and not stay for the PHP (partial) after that. We kept telling him to take it one step at a time. We had weekly counseling sessions with Zach and his counselor, and she said that he was doing great. When the 30 days was up, he agreed to stay for the PHP for a week, and then take it week by week after that. Every week, he asked to stay another week and before we knew it, eight weeks had gone by. As he progressed with the program, he was asked to mentor some of the newer people coming into the program. Here is where Zach found what he loved to do. He was born to be a counselor. He had so much experience with all that he had gone through, and he had also gone through so much counseling over the years. He had so much guidance to offer. He also was the most compassionate, nonjudgemental person I have ever known.

Over the years, he would go to many more inpatient treatment facilities, but Zach told me many years later, that La Ventana helped him the most. I think that was partially because he was asked to help other people who were struggling, and he discovered that he loved helping people. When we picked him up from the airport, he looked so healthy and he had the sparkle back in his eyes. I took a picture of him to capture that moment, and it's still one of my favorite pictures of him.

When he came home, he really had the bulimia under control, but a whole new set of problems arose. He now had severe stomach and digestive issues. This was clearly a result of the bulimia taxing his body, but I also felt that Zach's anxiety continued to manifest in different ways over the years: from severe OCD symptoms, to bulimia, to severe stomach issues, to substance abuse.

We went to see a gastroenterologist, which would be the first of many over the course of the next five years. He was prescribed various medications that usually didn't help at all. At one point, he was diagnosed with celiac disease, so he went on a gluten free diet. Later on he was told that he didn't have celiac (which was all quite confusing), but he remained on a GF diet almost all of the time, for the rest of his life. From that point forward, I made double dinners when we had pasta or bread crumbs. We discovered all of the GF breads and rolls and snacks that actually tasted good.

In the spring of 2015, things started to look brighter for Zach. He applied to the University of Buffalo for business and had been accepted for the fall semester. Even more importantly, he started dating Lily, who was the love of his life. She is a beautiful soul, quiet and gentle like Zach. They were a good match and he was really happy with her.

That summer, Zach and I went to the new student orientation at UB. I took a picture of him that day on his new campus and it was so surreal to be there with my son. It was hard to believe that I had gone there myself 25 years ago. Time really does fly by.

Fall came and it was Christopher's senior year and last year of football at Orchard Park High School. Our whole family was excited for another year of varsity football, especially Zach. When he stopped playing football, he completely immersed himself in his three brothers' high school sports careers. He was undoubtedly their biggest fan. He went to every game that he was able to. He even went to travel basketball games all over Western New York. I always loved having him as a companion at those games. All the parents and families knew Zach, and loved seeing his smiling face at the games. One of the basketball dads once said to me, "Zach is special, isn't he? He makes me happy just being around him." Yes. That was the truth right there.

Christopher had an amazing football season that year, even catching a touchdown pass at the championship game at the Bills stadium. It was so much fun for all of us. I remember that one of his coaches talked about him at the football banquet and said that when Christopher came onto the field, it was electrifying. I loved watching him play. Zach could not have been prouder of his boy.

Zach also started coaching Peter's Little Loop Football team with his dad. He absolutely loved it. He was always like the pied piper with kids; they adored him. I'm sure it was because he was so gentle and kind to all of them. He didn't judge the kids on their athletic ability at all and he treated all of them as equals (as it should be of course). The other parents and I would watch Zach from the stands as there was always a group of kids surrounding him on the sidelines. They were 12 and 13 year olds and they would talk to him incessantly, but Zach never lost his patience with them. He would just smile at them and nod. He always did prefer kids to adults.

All in all, on the surface, it seemed as though Zach was doing well. He was getting great grades at UB, working for his dad, and spending time with Lily. However, always below the surface, he struggled with his mental health. The OCD symptoms never went away, although his psychologist helped him to manage them.

CHAPTER NINE

I MUST DETOUR FROM Zach's story for a bit, because in January of 2016, a life changing event happened to me. My friend Lillian introduced me to a spiritual counselor/teacher named Jillian Greyse. Jillian is a passionate and knowledgeable transformational coach who has dedicated her life to empowering individuals to cultivate their intuition, personal power, and connection with their divine inner being. She believes that we all have the capacity to deepen our understanding of ourselves on a soul level. Her goal is to help individuals rediscover themselves and reclaim their inner power. I began working with her then, and have continued working with her ever since. I always say that she is my earth angel, but she always says that if I hadn't found her, I would have found someone else to help with my spiritual growth. Still, she was the one. She is my teacher.

It was perfect timing of course. Zach was not doing well, as often was the case in the winter months. It had been years of trying to help him and years of carrying sadness because he suffered. Keith and I had also gone through a really difficult breakup because of my complete lack of available free time, and I was definitely at a low point in my life. Jillian was living in Orchard Park at that time so I was able to do in person appointments. Zach even got to have several in person appointments with her as well. She has since moved out of state and does virtual appointments now. She has a YouTube channel and her email is jilliangreyse@gmail.com so please reach out if you're drawn to. I apologize in advance for the amount of times I will be mentioning her name throughout the rest of this book, however I sincerely feel that it is my responsibility to share the wisdom and knowledge that she has imparted to me.

Jillian has this amazing gift of getting you to see a situation in a different light, what we call reframing. One of the most important things I've learned in working with her is that we cannot take on other people's struggles, even if it happens to be our child. One of my life lessons in this life is for me to let go of trying to "save" or protect the ones I love. Every soul comes to earth to go through certain challenges in order to grow and advance spiritually. I had read in spiritual books that when we are souls on the "other side," we choose these challenges and situations that we will go through in this life on earth. We agree to them. Harry Jim once said to me, "Souls who choose to come to earth to go through mental illness are the bravest souls." I wholeheartedly agree with that. Of course I never ever said that to Zach, because that would have been cruel of me to insinuate that he chose to go through all that he had gone through.

Jillian continuously reminded me that this was Zach's journey and that I didn't have the right to take it on. Of course as his mom, it was my job to help him in every way possible, offering support and guiding him to professionals and spiritual teachers who could help him. However, what was not helpful was me "going down with the ship." For the past few years, I had felt like it was my JOB to be sad, depressed, and "down" whenever Zach was. Jillian helped me to see that this didn't help him at all, just as worrying about a situation doesn't help at all.

The only thing I could do, while supporting him, was to continue to work on myself; cultivating more self love, maintaining a daily spiritual practice, and monitoring my negative thoughts. It has been said that our thoughts create our world. Monitoring my negative thoughts has always been the most difficult thing for me. I have always been very hard on myself (an extreme perfectionist) and when I began really policing my thoughts, I realized how self sabotaging I had been for so long. Mantras have helped me tremendously with this, which I will talk about later on in the book.

For years, I had already had a daily yoga practice, even if some days it was only 15-20 minutes, and Jillian suggested that I start a daily meditation practice. Although it was difficult at first, after much practice, this became a game changer for me. For almost five years, I meditated every single morning.

Additionally, I began reiki training. It had been suggested to me in the past and I found a reiki I/II training in Western New York with a lovely woman through the International Center for Reiki Training. According to their website, "Reiki is a Japanese technique for stress reduction and relaxation that promotes healing. It is administered by 'laying on hands' and is based on the idea that an unseen 'life force energy' flows through us and is what causes us to be alive." It was a healing experience for me to go through the training. Six months later, I did the Master reiki training, and a year later, I did the Karuna Master training. Each training brought more healing to me. Reiki brought a deeper spirituality to the yoga classes I taught. I also began offering reiki sessions to clients. Most importantly, I started sending healing energy to Zach every day. I know it helped sometimes. Several times over the years when he was so severely depressed he couldn't get out of bed, I would sit in his room and send reiki to him, and later on, he would be downstairs watching sports with his brothers.

Spiritual work on ourselves is just that, so much WORK! I have been a work in progress for many years, as we all are. My friend Lillian always makes me laugh when we discuss our spiritual challenges; she always says, "Does it REALLY have to be so hard?" Nonetheless, the combination of reiki and daily yoga and meditation was what kept me balanced moving forward with all that we would continue to go through with Zach. Unfortunately, the road ahead would get progressively harder.

Winter and spring of 2016 was also an exciting time for Christopher and our family. It was his senior year basketball season, Senior Day for basketball, Senior prom, and high school graduation. Zach was present for all of it and if he was really struggling, he didn't admit it. I'm sure he did that for Christopher.

In May, I took my boys to Disney World for a long weekend. I had a Disney Visa card for many years and had accumulated a huge amount of Disney credit. This may not seem like a dream vacation to all moms, but to spend four days and nights with all of my boys was a dream for me. Even waiting in lines was quality time together. They are just pure fun. They always have fun together and that fun is contagious to be around. They are even patient with me when I want to see my favorite, Belle. I also was very melancholy, knowing that Christopher would be going away to college soon. Everything was about to change.

There is nothing Zach loved more than being around his brothers. He had a blast, even though his OCD was so extreme the morning we were leaving, we almost missed our flight because I couldn't get him out of the hotel room. All in all though, it was a great trip. There is a quote from Dr. Suess, *Sometimes you will never know the value of a moment, until it becomes a memory.* That would be the last vacation I would have with all of my boys.

That summer Zach worked as a counselor at the Y day camp for kids. This is where he really did shine. The kids just loved him. Even though he had just completed a year at UB for business, to me it was very clear that working with kids was his true calling. It fulfilled him. He considered changing his major, but the fact that he had three semesters of business classes under his belt deterred him.

Peter and I drove Christopher to college that summer. He was attending Mercyhurst University in Erie, Pennsylvania for business marketing. He decided to try out for the football team as a walk on, and he made the team. I was thrilled with his choice since it was an experience away from home like he wanted, but it was only an hour and half drive which meant lots of visits! I was very emotional when we left him because I was going to miss him so much, but I was thankful that it was nothing like dropping Zach off at Duquesne. Christopher was ready and eager to start his new adventure, and that is all a parent can hope for. Fortunately for me, he would pop home for a weekend visit every month since it was so close. He loved to surprise me and just appear at my door. Nothing better.

CHAPTER TEN

ZACH HAD ALWAYS been somewhat private about all of his struggles with mental health. He didn't try to hide it, but he wasn't very open about it either. That summer when he was 20 years old, everything changed. He began to use social media as a platform for talking about his severe obsessive-compulsive disorder and anxiety and depression. At first his dad and I were uncomfortable with it. Back then, mental health was not talked about so openly as it is today and we worried that Zach would be ridiculed or bullied. Zach, however, never cared or worried about that.

What was important to him was sharing his story so that it might help someone else who was struggling with mental health issues to feel less isolated, to know that they are not alone with their struggles. We wouldn't find out until many years later how many people he truly helped with his posts. Zach was viewed as a handsome, intelligent, super nice guy that everyone loved. When he began to share the truth of all that he had gone through, and continued to go through, in such a raw and honest way, it really demonstrated that you can't judge a book by it's cover. From the outside, Zach appeared to have the "perfect" life, and yet he suffered greatly. People he barely knew have told me that his honesty helped them realize they were not alone. Putting himself out there in such a vulnerable way took so much courage. I am so proud of his bravery and selflessness to try and help others. I believe that Zach was a trailblazer back then, leading the way for people to be as open and honest as he was about mental health. In July of 2016, Zach wrote an essay about his life with OCD on a platform called Stigma Fighters:

STIGMA FIGHTERS: ZACH LIBERATORE

Hello my name is Zach Liberatore and I am a victim of Obsessive-Compulsive Disorder. I was clinically diagnosed with it and prescribed medication during the end of 2012 when I checked into the psychiatric ward at ECMC. This disease dragged me to the brink of insanity and I had reached the point where I no longer wanted to live. I seriously contemplated suicide because I could never get away from the tormenting thoughts and the compulsions that came along with them. Most of the opportunities I have blown throughout these recent years were due to my inability to control and fight the disease. I began to ingest drugs and alcohol thinking it would alleviate the symptoms; it turns out they only made things worse in the long run. I've ruined close friendships because I was no longer able to hang out with people without being consumed by these thoughts and compulsions. I've cried up to roughly one thousand times because I'd feel so alone and dejected. The world's lack of understanding for our disease is sickening because it truly does deteriorate our well-being and suicides often occur because of it. It's time for us to start sharing our experiences and battles with mental illness in order to give society a better understanding of the cruelty and torture that comes along with mental disorders.

I have experienced thousands of different symptoms regarding the disease, consequently making it incredibly difficult for me to list every single one. But I can inform you of some of my most traumatic and disturbing experiences and symptoms. One incident I typically resort to telling occurred during the winter of 2012, the event which triggered the idea to enter a psychiatric ward. After being completely worn down from the thoughts and urges throughout a week during this winter, I decided to take a stroll into the woods behind my grandfather's house. I felt as if it'd bring satisfaction and would maybe relieve the overwhelming distress. It had been snowing all week so I dressed up appropriately and set foot into the woods. Looking back I believe I travelled up to two miles into the woods without looking back. After being in there for a significant amount of time, I decided it was time to return home. Along the way into the woods I had obviously made plenty of footsteps in the snow; this instantly triggered an obsessive thought. Even though it's utterly irrational, my mind kept reiterating to walk backwards to my house and place my feet into every footstep previously made or I couldn't leave. It sounds crazy but this essentially summarizes my life with OCD. I couldn't even make it past the first few steps because I never felt satisfied with how my feet placed into the initial footsteps. I could've miraculously placed my foot perfectly but I still wouldn't be content. I spent up to four hours in those woods, crying and considering the pain that would go away if I were to kill myself.

This incident was only one of many experiences that triggered a loss for hope. I received exceptional grades throughout my life and was always motivated to do well in the academic field. When the OCD came upon me, my grades and motivation level progressively decreased. A lot of my symptoms were number oriented and I began to only rely on four numbers: 9 (which was for my mother), 7 (which was for my youngest brother), 5 (which was for my other two brothers between the youngest and me), and 8 (which was for my father). Anytime I used a number that was not 9,7,5 or 8, I would feel as if I was disrespecting my family and that even something tragic would happen to one of them. Even though I knew the correct answers for math tests, I would fail the tests because I wouldn't be able to use any number besides those four. Writing and reading became huge issues which both directly impacted my grades. I could no longer take notes in class because it would take me up to an hour to write one letter. There wasn't a specific way the letter had to be written, I was just never content with how I had written it. I would fail tests in every other subject because I wouldn't be able to complete the essays and short answer questions. Whenever I was assigned a reading assignment I could not finish one line on a page because for every word, I had to say each letter out loud in my head then proceed to tell myself the definition of the word. This may not even seem so horrible but the thoughts would then transition into believing I didn't say the letter the right way in my head, or I was pausing while telling myself the definitions.

I've nearly been in numerous car accidents due to OCD affecting how I drive. Everything I did, not just driving, had to be symmetric no matter what. I would touch something with my right hand and then proceed to touch it with my left. I'd shake someone's hand and then make up a lame excuse to shake their hand with my opposite hand. There are far more examples but I want to primarily focus on the driving. When driving down a certain road, the idea of symmetry would suddenly pop up in my mind. There-fore, my mind would tell me to drive across the double yellow line into the other lane. I would have to do it as soon as I was told which clearly would be an issue with incoming vehicles approaching. Anytime I saw a bump or crack in the road, or even the sidewalk, I would get the urge to run it over. If I had failed to do so, I would quickly turn my car around to do it. I noticed bumps or cracks on sidewalks and would sometimes drive onto the sidewalks just to run them over. It would take me hours to go to a friend's house or even school.

One of my most recent symptoms has been revolved around hurting or torturing animals and even insects. I know it's irrational to believe that insects have complex brains and should be treated as humans or animals, but it doesn't matter because my brain tells me this is how it is. I do landscaping for my father during summers which includes mulching and mowing lawns. Very often I would put mulch over an ant or a worm and would get tremen-dously distraught. Sometimes I would finish mulching a certain bed of soil then frantically dig through it in order to find the ant or worm I put it over. Rocks are commonly present in or on beds of soil which became another signif-icant problem. Even though it'd be totally evident that it's just a rock, I would firmly believe I had just put soil over an animal and it was suffering. Mowing lawns was the same deal; I'd run over a bottle, piece of clothing, rock, etc., and my mind would tell me that I had just run over an animal. After finishing a lawn, I'd navigate the whole lawn to see if there was a suffering animal. The same is-sue occurs while I'm driving, so I am constantly turning around on every road I drive on just to see if I had indeed run over an animal.

Like I've previously stated, these are only a couple of symptoms out of the thousands that I have dealt with for the past six years. OCD is usually misconstrued as an adjective in which people use to describe their neat and clean tendencies. I'm sure there are plenty of people who deal with the same symptoms as I do and take great offense to how often the term "OCD" is tossed around. I'm not going to lie and say this is a cake walk battling the OCD, but I also do not do this often: telling people my story or symptoms. I did not write this to expect sympathy; I wrote it to reach out to the thousands of children and adults who unfortunately must battle the same disease on a daily basis. I wrote this in order to help these intrepid and lionhearted people understand that they are not alone, that they are not freaks. People need to start speaking up as I just did in writing this essay so the world becomes better educated on the disease and will hopefully begin to show a little more empathy for it. This disease has tormented my life the past six years: ruining friendships, opening the door for drugs and causing too much emotional torture and anguish. I will continue fighting this mental battle because I know I'm strong enough and I know I have the support of family, friends and God; I will not let it commandeer my life. In conclusion, I'd like to reach out to the millions of people who struggle with OCD around the globe. This battle is one of the most distressful and hurtful experiences you'll deal with in your lifetime. It will bring you to your knees, begging God or another higher power to take away the pain. You will debate with yourself whether or not you would like to continue living. In these times of discomfort and agony, consider this: defeating this plague will only make you stronger. God chooses his strongest soldiers to fight the biggest battles. Never give up because the world needs you and your perseverance. One day you'll have full and utter control of the disease and will be able to help others who are just beginning the horrible journey. The people who are skeptical of our struggles and the disease itself are just blind to the capabilities and power of the human brain. Reach out and speak up about your disease because it will only help. Be strong and whether you believe in God or not, know there is some sort of higher power that has your back through it all.

 ZACH LIBERATORE
 20 YEARS OLD
 BUFFALO, NY

We never saw that essay back when Zach posted it on Stigma Fighters. Most people he knew probably didn't follow Stigma Fighters or see the essay, however I'm sure he helped many people who did see it. When we did see it was almost four years later when he posted the essay on his Facebook page. I was blown away by his essay; it was so raw and honest and brave. I shared it, as well as over a hundred other people and the response back then, as well as every time it is shared, is incredible. He has helped so many people understand what OCD really is. He has helped countless people who struggle with OCD and other mental health challenges feel understood and less alone. He could not have imagined when he wrote this, the impact that it would have, and continues to have. It truly shows how one act of bravery can make such a difference in the world. I am so proud of him.

In the fall of 2016, he posted on Facebook:

> *After almost 4 years of going to the Children's Psychiatric Clinic, I am just about finished. The people there have helped tremendously and I recommend it to anyone experiencing mental health issues. Get the help you need ASAP!*

(He thought that he would be aging out at 21, but fortunately he was able to continue on.) This post was probably a shock to many people who did not know that Zach struggled with mental illness, or that he had been seeing both a psychologist and psychiatrist for four years. This was really when he let his guard down and began his crusade to break the stigma of mental illness. He always encouraged people to share their stories, and to never be ashamed to get the help they needed. Whether we were ready for it or not, our family was thrust into the spotlight of mental health. We always supported Zach in his efforts to reach out to people who were suffering.

Shortly after that, he posted:

> *For most of us, all we've had is ourselves. Lets try to change that for everyone battling mental illness today and in the future. #BellsLetsTalk*

Bell Let's Talk Day was an initiative to promote public discussions around mental health. It put a spotlight on mental illness and the hashtag #BellsLetsTalk on Twitter was tweeted by millions of people to show solidarity and prevent stigma for those who suffer from depression, OCD, and other anxiety disorders. Zach was proud to be part of that movement.

In the meantime, life went on with our boys in school and sports. That fall, Peter's Little Loop team won the championship for his last year (and our family's last year) of Little Loop football. Zach, Christopher and Eric were so proud and loved watching their little brother play football. It was the end of an era for us. We had spent fourteen years at Little Loop games.

That December, we celebrated Zach's 21st birthday. No matter how old my boys are, we always celebrate their birthday with birthday cake with our whole family, including their grandparents and aunts. As Zach continued to struggle every year, his birthday was always bittersweet for him and for us. We celebrated that he was with us for another year and we had hope of better quality of life in the year ahead, but there was always the underlying sadness of how difficult his life was.

When my boys were little and I thought ahead to the day that each of them would turn 21, officially an adult, I imagined how wonderful and exciting their lives would be. No amount of spiritual work on myself, not yoga or meditation or breathing techniques, could change the fact that I wanted my boy to have a happy life. Yes I knew it was his journey but as his mom, I hurt when he hurt. There is a saying that goes, "A mother is only as happy as her unhappiest child." Any parent who has a child who suffers understands this to be true. Yet, our spiritual teachers tell us that this is not how it should be. It is our job to be happy from within, and not have our happiness determined by outside factors, even if that factor happens to be our child. It was an ongoing work in progress for me. I always told Zach that all I ever wanted for him was to be happy and at peace.

CHAPTER ELEVEN

THE WINTER OF 2017 marked the beginning of Eric's varsity basketball career. Eric excelled at basketball and it brought our entire family joy to watch him play. Zach was the quintessential proud big brother to all of his brothers and he was sure that each one of them was always THE BEST player on their team. No one could tell him otherwise.

You may not know that in a high school football season there is typically one game per week, but for basketball there can be two or even three games a week. Zach was at almost every game with us, whether home or away.

Eric had a really exciting season, and even made the Orchard Park High School record book by making 13 assists in one game, which was the second most assists in a game in OPHS history! He was a point guard, lightning fast, but my favorite thing about Eric as a basketball player was that he was as humble and gracious on the court as he is in life.

Zach spent time going to Eric's games, as well as Peter's games at his school, plus both of their travel games, while he was still a student at UB and worked at the Y. He was also still in a relationship with Lily. He was busy with life, but always had his ups and downs, good days and bad.

2017 was a big year of change for our family in many ways. I sold the house that we had lived in for 24 years. It had become too expensive for me to maintain and I had put it on the market the previous year with no luck. After thirty house showings in which I had to have the house immaculate with boys and dog out of the house, it finally sold. I bought a smaller house in another neighborhood in Orchard Park and it even has a yoga room separate from the rest of the house where I take clients.

This was difficult for all of us. It was the house that all of my boys grew up in, the house where they took their first steps, and spoke their first words. It was a beautiful home where most of my boys' memories were made and it was sad for us to say goodbye to it.

Fate may have stepped in to make the transition easier for us. Two weeks before closing, the master bathtub which hadn't worked in ten years, suddenly sprang to life. A blocked pipe must have been cleared and someone must have turned the faucet on during an inspection, so the water ran for several hours, filling up the bathtub and then overflowing into the bedroom and leaking into the kitchen underneath, ruining all the hardwood floors. It was a disaster.

My stress was through the roof, trying to pack up twenty four years worth of stuff and manage the insurance claim and clean up the house all at once. It was a $100,000 mess. It certainly made it easier for us to leave the house after weeks of living in a complete mess. Still, it was a very difficult day as we said goodbye to our first home.

At the same time, Peter and I were both in serious relationships that affected the boys for the first time ever. Melissa had moved into Peter's house and Keith was spending a lot of time at our new house. Peter graduated from 8th grade and was about to start high school. All of our boys were busy with their friends and their own lives so Peter and I both had free time to begin more permanent relationships.

All of this change was inevitably hard for Zach, being someone who struggled with change, as well as dealing with his stomach issues and OCD symptoms with additional people around, even though Keith and Melissa became part of the family. Zach talked about getting an apartment. It was too financially difficult for him since he was still in school, however the real reason I believe he never moved out was because he needed us as his support system. Peter and I were definitely in agreement that we preferred having him at home so that we could keep an eye on him. At least we knew he was safe.

Somewhere along the way Zach began to self medicate. We had certainly been warned by more than one counselor that this could happen. All of the medications that he was prescribed over the years, from Zoloft to Xanax to Klonopin and Hydroxyzine, never did take away his severe OCD symptoms and depression. He began experimenting with other pills such as Valium and Oxycodone. Eventually Opana would be his painkiller of choice. All of these would numb the pain temporarily.

We wouldn't find out about it until years later. It wasn't constant at first; just on occasions when he just couldn't take the OCD anymore. He was afraid of getting addicted; for years I had lectured him and all of my boys on how easy it was to get addicted to painkillers. He also began to drink more and I think it was his fear of getting addicted to the pills that made him choose alcohol instead.

We began what would become a rollercoaster of ups and downs with Zach. He was either severely depressed spending all of his time in his room or at the other end of the spectrum, he would go out with friends, get very drunk and often not come home and not respond to texts. There was no in between. For Peter and me, it was utterly exhausting and now even more than before, it was affecting his brothers as well as Keith and Melissa.

Yet, there was always this dichotomy with Zach. He would drive us crazy, drinking and getting into trouble, but then his true personality would shine through and we would get the loveliest of compliments about him. For example, there was his first arrest. (Not a proud mom moment.) There is an outdoor concert venue near us called Darien Lake. They sell a huge amount of lawn seats to young people and many of them drink alcohol before the concert. Zach went with his friends to the first concert of the season and was kicked out by security because they were drinking. He made the moronic decision to jump the fence and go back in and he was arrested with a whole slew of young people.

When his dad went to pick him up from the Darien jail, the woman who released him told Peter that "Out of the 100 kids arrested, Zach is the nicest prisoner we have ever had." Anyone who knows Zach would laugh at that because you just know that it's true. For this mama bear, it wasn't funny at the time that my first born child had been arrested. (Although I did just laugh out loud while I was writing that story.) As always, he was grounded and he was sincerely sorry that he had messed up. As usual, depression ensued because he felt like he had disappointed us.

A week later, an Orchard Park mom posted a picture on Zach's Face-book page of Zach and her 12 year old son at the Y and she wrote:

> *Why I love the Y... because of awesome people like Mr.*
> *Zach. My son ran into him, not even working today, but*
> *Zach still willingly hung out with my 10 yr old for about*
> *an hour! I hope nothing more than to raise young men just*
> *like Mr. Zach, what a nice kid. My boys are so lucky to have*
> *fantastic role models!*

No matter what he was going through in his life, Zach was kind and generous to people, and I will always be proud of him for that.

In fall of 2017, Peter began his freshman year of high school, Eric began his senior year of high school and Christopher went back to Mercyhurst for sophomore year of college. While Eric and Peter were enjoying all the fun activities of Fall Homecoming, Zach went downhill. His depression got worse. His stomach issues got worse. He was diagnosed with IBS (irritable bowl syndrome). He told me that his depression was so bad he couldn't even hang out with his friends. He sent me this text:

> *I'm just really depressed and I'm thinking horrible things.*
> *And honestly I've been drinking a lot and doing Adderall*
> *and its all messing with my head. And I just feel like I'm at*
> *the lowest point of my life.*

As my other sons were busy with high school and college and sports and their friends, my oldest son was feeling like he was at the lowest point of his life at the age of 21. He thought about suicide again. He went to Brylin inpatient again for a week and it was right in the middle of the semester, so he didn't finish the semester. He was thinking about changing his major to become a teacher or mental health counselor.

Shortly after Zach was released from Brylin, Keith and I had a trip planned to go to Aspen, Colorado to visit his brother. I was on the fence as to whether I should still go, but Zach insisted he was doing better and wanted me to go. Unbeknownst to me, Keith was planning on proposing on the trip and had wanted to tell my boys before we left, however with all that Zach had been going through, he did not feel that it was right to tell them. We did get engaged at 12,000 feet at Independence Pass and had a wonderful trip, even though a part of me felt guilty for being happy when my Zach was not. I was still working on that "I can only be as happy as my unhappiest child" thing. I struggled with the underlying sadness. We told the boys when we got home and they were all happy that I was happy. Keith officially moved in.

In December, we celebrated Zach's 22nd birthday. He also talked to his advisor at UB and changed his major to Health and Human Services. Although he would now be even further from graduating because he had taken so many business classes, at least he was excited about his future. This gave me hope.

CHAPTER TWELVE

2018 WAS THE YEAR that everything got worse than it already had been; the beginning of the downward spiral for Zach. Two life changing events happened to him in early 2018.

Zach's psychologist at the Children's Psychiatric Clinic that he had been with for five years told us that Zach had aged out from the clinic. He had thought that he could continue for another year, but the rules of insurance would not allow it. This was quite a blow for Zach. He had helped Zach tremendously and Zach depended on him to get through really difficult times. I know that it affected him more than he let on.

Even more devastating for Zach was that he and Lily broke up. I cannot comment on the details of their relationship, but I know that it was completely Zach's fault. He was not in a good place and he did not treat Lily as she deserved to be treated. I am sure that she stayed with him longer than she should have, but she loved him. I know that she remained in his life after that, they talked every day, and Zach always held onto hope that when he was better, he and Lily would get back together. I think she felt the same way. I always thought that someday they would get married and have a family. As I said before, she was the love of his life. I know that she has struggled with his death, but she has absolutely no reason to have guilt.

While all of that was happening with Zach, life went on with my other boys. It was Eric's senior basketball season and Peter's freshman basketball season and all of their games were back to back, both home and away. We all went to every game of course, including Zach.

Eric had an incredible season. One of their games was against their big rival Jamestown High School which was an hour and half drive away. A mom once said to me that she envied how close my boys were, and loved how they always supported one another by going to each other's games. I hadn't really thought about it that much, but that night as I took a photo of Zach and Christopher together, who had each driven an hour and half on a weeknight (Zach from Buffalo and Christopher from Erie) to watch their younger brothers play high school basketball games, I really appreciated how they supported each other. I felt very blessed at that moment. It had been fourteen years since Orchard Park had beaten Jamestown in Jamestown, and that night Orchard Park won. It was really exciting and fun.

Eric's team made it to the playoffs at Buffalo State College and once again Christopher drove up from college to be there. After Eric's last high school game, I took a picture of the four of them on the court. I love the complete look of happiness on Eric's face and the pride on his brothers' faces.

As all of this was going on, I had a feeling that Zach was drinking more. This was confirmed on a trip that we all took to Disney World. Peter had made the Buffalo Bills Flag Football team and they were competing in a tournament at the Pro Bowl in Disney World. Of course none of us were going to miss this! The entire family went: Keith and me, Peter and Melissa, Zach and Christopher. Eric had to stay behind because he had basketball.

Even though Zach and Christopher were often on their own, I could tell Zach was sneaking drinks on this trip and to make matters worse, his psychologist had put him on Xanax so he was mixing Xanax with alcohol. It was difficult to enjoy the trip worrying about Zach and knowing that he was not in a good place and headed down a bad path.

Not long after that, Zach was arrested for speeding and reckless driving and his car was impounded. He was not intoxicated, but it was one more thing to take care of. Peter picked him up from jail and I had to bring Zach back to pay to get his car back. He had to go to court for multiple charges and his dad generously hired an attorney we knew to represent Zach. He was released with a fine. As always, when Zach disrupted our lives, he was filled with guilt afterward and then that led to depression. It was a vicious cycle.

Around that time, Peter and I began seeing a family counselor named Bob, recommended by a friend. We needed some guidance on how to handle all of the "Zach stuff" while also keeping a healthy environment for our other boys. No easy task, but he was really helpful for us. He asked for Zach to come to some of the appointments, which he did.

Bob had solid advice which we followed, including having Zach work for his dad to help pay for the attorney and cost of his arrest. Even though Zach's drinking had escalated, he did not recommend forcing him to move out of our homes. Every counselor, psychologist and psychiatrist were still in agreement; with his severe OCD and history of suicidal thoughts, forcing him out away from his family could very well be a death sentence.

That March, I got a text from Zach:

I have a drinking problem.

We talked at length and he disclosed how much he had been drinking. I was grateful that at least he admitted it and wanted to get help. He began going to a substance abuse counselor at Horizon Health Services. Obviously mixing alcohol with all of the prescribed medications he was taking was extremely dangerous and it was difficult to not be in a constant state of worry. In addition to the yoga classes and clients I was teaching, I took on a second job as a receptionist at a local day spa, so I was very busy which kept my mind occupied.

That Easter, Keith and the boys and I were invited down to visit our friends Patty and Pete in Charlotte, NC. Pete worked for the Charlotte Hornets NBA team at that time, so the plan was to take the boys to an NBA game on Easter along with their son. Zach opted not to go because he didn't want to miss any classes and had a lot of work to do for school.

We were having a wonderful weekend when just as we were getting ready to leave for the game, I got a call from Zach's dad. Zach had been taken to ECMC. He had been with friends and accidentally overdosed on his Klonopin. He was stable and was going to be fine, but would be in the hospital for a few days. It was not a suicide attempt. He said that his OCD thoughts were debilitating and he was trying to get some relief.

I didn't know what to do. I wanted to skip the game and drive the ten hours home to see Zach. At the same time, I didn't want to ruin my boys' trip. Peter was adamant; Zach was going to be okay and he was asleep at the hospital so he insisted that we go to the game and dinner as planned and drive back in the morning.

If I had been alone, I would have gone home to be with Zach, but I wanted my boys to be able to enjoy the day. So much of their lives had revolved around Zach for so long. Peter and I tried our best to make them a priority but the focus of the family always went back to Zach. Christopher, Eric and Peter NEVER ever complained about it. They loved their big brother so much and they just wanted him to be healthy and happy.

So off to the game we went. The boys all sat courtside and hung out in the VIP lounge. It was a great day for everyone, but for me it was difficult to relax and have fun when my boy was in the hospital. For so many years, my worry for Zach was like background music that was always playing. It was impossible to escape. Everyone had fun until dinner when Eric had shrimp for the first time and had an allergic reaction, his throat closing up. The manager gave him Benadryl, so crisis averted thank God, but never a dull moment!

I went directly to the hospital when we got home and Zach was already heading deep into depression again. The psychiatrist he used to see at the Children's Psychiatric Clinic was on call at ECMC and he had always had a soft spot for Zach (as everyone always did). He suggested that Peter and I be in charge of his Klonopin from that point forward.

When he got home, Zach admitted that he needed a higher level of care to deal with his drinking problem, so we began to research inpatient facilities for substance abuse. He had heard of Conifer Park near Albany, NY and was referred by a friend who went there, so Zach did the intake and was accepted. As he prepared to leave, he wrote on his Facebook page:

I owe my parents the world.

CHAPTER THIRTEEN

In May of 2018, I drove Zach to yet another inpatient facility. It was a five hour drive and I planned on driving immediately back after going through the intake procedure with him. This was a very different experience from any of the treatment facilities he had been to. My involvement would be minimal. Zach signed papers, I was given paperwork and told that he would not be allowed to have his phone at all, and there would be no family involvement or counseling. He would be able to call home from the house phone at designated times. They asked me to take all of his money; he wasn't allowed to have any.

I think I was there for all of twenty minutes and then it was time for me to go. We hugged goodbye.

I said, "Everything will be okay. Love you."

"Bye mom. Love you too."

It didn't feel right leaving him there. He was an adult but he was only 22 after all. This was a facility filled with grown men. I cried as I walked out and prayed, "God, please heal my Zach."

It was an AA 12-step program and he was there for 30 days. There were no issues with him asking to leave; he followed the program perfectly. He sounded good on his calls to us, however he talked at length about how most of the men there had serious alcohol and drug addiction, in and out of rehab for years. He met heroin addicts who had served time and were sent there directly from prison. It seemed a little hardened for Zach, but I tried to stick to my mantra, "Everything happens for a reason" and figured maybe this was all good for Zach. Perhaps he would see that this could be his future if he didn't manage it now.

He was sent home on a bus for a six hour drive with no money, just a bag lunch. I remember that when I pulled up to the Buffalo bus station to pick him up, he looked older, more mature. He didn't want to talk much about it, but I'm sure that being in group counseling all day, every day with drug addicts and reformed criminals was very eye opening for this boy who grew up in suburban Orchard Park. I think he grew up a lot that month.

He was proud of himself for completing the 30 days. He was given a gold sobriety coin that he kept on his dresser from that point on. He had a box of letters, written from men he had met while he was there, letters of encouragement for when he was released. It was then that I realized how such strong bonds were formed between people in treatment, in such a short amount of time. They bared their souls in group counseling and exposed their lives to complete strangers. These men got to know the real Zach very well, and they loved and admired him. Some wrote that he had encouraged and helped them. All of them wrote that he spoke of his family often and with love, and that he wanted more than anything to make us proud.

One letter in particular stood out. A young man wrote:

> Zach, I honestly think you were one of the first people I've ever opened up to, and I have no idea why. I honestly have never met anybody your age, or any age, that's ever made me feel so comfortable. I've never told anybody the stuff I told you man.

We would continue to hear that for years to come. Zach was a natural born counselor.

He also wrote:

*Be that role model you've always wanted to be for your
brothers. Be that son your parents think so highly of.*

I always wrote Zach a letter when he was going to an inpatient, telling him how proud I was of him and how strong and courageous he was. When I recently went through his desk at home, I found that he had kept all of those letters. He also kept the cards and letters that Francine had sent him at Conifer park, as well as a letter his dad had written him when he left. He always really did want to make all of us proud, especially his brothers.

He was home just in time for Eric's AAU basketball team competing in the National Championship in Ohio. We didn't know if this was the best idea for him to immediately travel with us, but there was no arguing with Zach over this; he was going to watch his boy play. Thank goodness he came because Eric's team made it to the championship game and won the whole thing!

Eric had started playing with this team when he was 16. "Coach Mike" as they called him, hand picked his players from all over Western New York and he recruited Eric to be on the team. I clearly remember taking Eric to the initial meeting of the team. As coach Mike was explaining the demands of the team, the rigorous practice schedule all over WNY, the games across states, and the fact that we had no one to carpool with because Eric was the only kid from Orchard Park, I was thinking to myself "No way. There is no way he is doing this." I had three boys in sports in addition to all that we went through with Zach. I looked over at Eric and he never looked so excited about anything in his life. Of course we would do this for Eric.

It turned out to be one of our smartest decisions. Not only did this team help mold Eric into the basketball player he was, he also forged deep bonds and friendships with coach Mike and his teammates. How fun was it for our family to watch these games and to be there to see Eric's team win the championship! Eric had an incredible game, one of the best games of his life. I miss watching that boy play basketball. After the game, Zach asked me to take a picture of Eric and him. The pride on Zach's face melts my heart.

A week later was Eric's high school graduation. When we were researching residential inpatient facilities, Zach had been adamant. He would not go anywhere that would prohibit him from getting to Eric's high school graduation. Fortunately, he had immediately gotten in to Conifer Park, so it all worked out. We took a family photo of Peter and me with our four boys after the ceremony. That was the last photo taken of the six of us. We went out for a graduation dinner with the entire family and it was so nice to have Zach there.

We had hoped that Zach would continue a sober lifestyle, but we also knew how difficult this was going to be for a 22 year old in summer in Buffalo with his friends who all drank. Summer in Buffalo is glorious but short. All of the outdoor concerts, beach bars, outdoor patios, and festivals are squeezed into a few months and it's a lot of fun for young people especially.

Zach tried sobriety, at first attending AA meetings, and then he attempted to drink "only socially and responsibly" which led to us being in a constant state of worry once again, especially since he was on so many medications for OCD and stomach issues. From that point forward, I never kept any liquor in the house and if we had wine, I hid it. We rarely had wine anymore at family dinners or holidays because I didn't want Zach to feel left out and didn't want to encourage drinking. Peter and I continued to monitor his Klonopins. We made it clear that drinking was not a good idea for him and obviously drinking and driving was off limits. If it ever happened, we would take the car away.

The years that followed became even more difficult. If Zach was being social and going out with friends, he was drinking, and I had to work very hard on myself to not be in a constant state of worry. I continued my daily yoga and meditation practice which helped me stay sane and somewhat balanced. It was around that time that I began a daily gratitude practice. For years, I had done gratitude journals on and off, but I began a simple routine of just beginning and ending each day with what I was grateful for. Very often it was something as simple as, "My boys are all safe and alive."

I also used mantras to calm my mind down when I started to worry about Zach. A mantra is a spiritual phrase or positive affirmation. It helps to have a "go to" mantra that you can repeat to yourself when your brain chatter gets going. My main mantra is: "Everything is exactly as it's supposed to be. Or it wouldn't be." "All is well" is another good one. Sometimes I would chant them in a loop when I was really stressed about Zach.

If Zach was drinking, he often wouldn't respond to texts because he wouldn't want us to know that he was drinking, and of course we would have no idea where he was or if he was okay. One Saturday night (of many), I hadn't seen or heard from him all night and I texted him the next morning:

Please text me that you're alive Zach.

He responded at noon:

I'm alive.

I was not being flippant. If he didn't respond to texts, it meant that he was drinking on top of his OCD meds plus Klonopin. Not to mention, alcohol is a depressant; so for a boy who already struggled with depression, we knew that drinking on medications could lead to extreme suicidal thoughts and possibly suicide.

For Peter and me, this was at the back of our minds for eight years. There was always the terrifying reality that he could take his own life. If he wasn't going out with friends, he was in his room in a deep state of depression, lying in bed in the dark or watching episode after episode of *The Office* on his laptop. His OCD obsessive thoughts would get the best of him and his bulimia was back full force. It was difficult to get him to come down for dinner or even get him out of the house for one of Peter's games. He would spend half the time in the bathroom and half the time in his room all day and all night. He either took five showers a day, or went five days without a shower.

For Peter and me, there was nothing worse than seeing our boy like this. It was difficult when he would be out with friends and we were worrying, but this was much, much worse. This was not living. This was not quality of life. We continued to get him help. I know that there are many people with mental health struggles and/or addiction that give up sometimes on going for counseling, but Zach never did. Even on his darkest days, he was always fighting to get better, fighting to live. That is why I always told him he was a warrior and that he was the strongest person I knew. He never gave up. He continued going to his psychologist, psychiatrist, and addiction counselor, but he spiraled downward again in the fall of 2018. He was suicidal and asked us to take him to Brylin inpatient again to "keep him safe."

He spent almost a week there but when he got home, he wasn't doing any better and a month after he had been released, he asked to go back to Brylin. He spent Thanksgiving there. It was sad for me to have Thanksgiving dinner without him, but I tried not to show it in front of my other boys and my family. Peter and I were always diligent about making sure our boys didn't miss out on anything because of Zach, but they surely struggled inwardly about the well being of their big brother. I can't imagine how hard it was for them to always carry that worry.

Meanwhile we tried to keep their lives as normal as possible. Christopher was still at Mercyhurst, Eric had started college at SUNY Erie, and Peter was in his sophomore year of high school. Peter was excelling at football and basketball and Zach went to most of his games with us when he could.

We headed into the holiday season and Zach's 23rd birthday with heavy hearts because Zach was no better. Unbelievably, he not only finished his semester at UB, while missing two solid weeks of school to go to Brylin, but he even made the Dean's List! I thought that this was incredibly impressive and Zach was proud of himself.

He continued to get worse instead of better. OCD obsessions and compulsions took over his days, he was throwing up his food constantly, and he had severe stomach pain all the time. By this point he was on OCD meds (I believe it was Zoloft at that time), Klonopin, plus Linzesse, Miralax, Gas X, and laxatives for all of his stomach and digestive issues. No wonder he had stomach issues. His life was a nightmare.

CHAPTER FOURTEEN

In January of 2019, Zach was at Peter's house, distraught and crying and texting me. When Peter walked into his room, he had a razor blade and was scraping at his wrist. We don't believe that he was trying to take his life; he could have done it if he wanted to. This was another cry for help. We took him back to Brylin. I prayed, "God, please heal my Zach." This time he was there for my birthday.

All I wanted for my birthday was to be with all four of my sons, so Christopher, Eric and Peter all came with me to visit Zach. We had to sneak two of them in because only two visitors were allowed, and Peter was not the required 18 and older. I am usually a rule follower, but I felt strongly that this was an occasion when rules were meant to be broken. It was the first time the boys had ever visited Zach at an inpatient facility. In the past, Zach had never wanted them to see him there.

We sat in a room with a bunch of other patients and their visitors. We just sat at a table and talked while Zach's brothers made him laugh as they always did. I remember being so filled with gratitude at that moment, so grateful to be with all four of my boys on my birthday, and so grateful that Zach was alive.

It became apparent that Zach was Mr. Popular at Brylin. This had become his "safe" place and he was very comfortable there. The staff loved him and all the patients loved him. He went out of his way to flash his Zach smile at each person, and when they talked to him, he would give them the Zach nod; in that nod was patience, compassion, empathy, non-judgement, and sincerity all at once. Everyone who knew Zach, knew that nod. He had a way of making you feel heard and understood. Everyone loved Zach. He would have been an amazing counselor.

When he was released, it was suggested that he needed an intensive outpatient program (IOP) and he was going to be starting the ECMC IOP for mental health. It was all day, everyday for a week and worked out well because UB would start as soon as it ended. On day three, I got a call from Zach that his good friend Joe had been brought into the ER at ECMC. He had been in a bad car accident and was fighting for his life. Zach spent that week going to the IOP and then sitting with Joe at the same hospital. He sent me a picture of his hand on Joe's hand. It was reminiscent of Nolan. It looked as though Zach could lose another friend, but the reverse would happen. Miraculously, Joe made it through and even though at one point Zach said that he may never walk again, Joe beat all the odds and is doing amazingly well!

Zach was back at UB, but we felt like we were watching a train wreck in slow motion. He was either out with friends and we wouldn't see him for days, or he was locked in his room or the bathroom. Bulimia had taken over his life again. By March, he admitted that he needed a higher level of care and asked to do another eating disorder inpatient program. He didn't want to drop out of UB mid semester and be pushed even further behind, but he knew that he had no choice. He needed help immediately.

Once again it was difficult to find an eating disorder inpatient treatment facility that took adult males and had an immediate bed available. We were referred to a place in North Carolina and Zach did the intake and they had a bed available immediately, so in March, Zach got on a plane to North Carolina. He insisted that he go alone this time since he was an adult and it was his third inpatient stay. I hugged him goodbye.

"Everything will be okay. Love you."

"Bye mom. Love you too."

I prayed, "God, please heal my Zach."

Sadly, whenever Zach went to an inpatient treatment facility, it was a bit of a relief for Peter and me. While there was always the background worry about Zach, for that brief period we knew that he was safe and he was getting help and we could focus completely on our other sons. This time however, was not the case. It was a disaster from start to finish.

The first week was a nightmare. Zach texted and called every day when he had his phone that he was in severe stomach pain. First the dietician insisted that he was not gluten intolerant enough to warrant a GF diet (even though he had been previously diagnosed as gluten intolerant), so he suddenly had gluten in his diet after years of being gluten free. I was calling back and forth for days between the treatment center and his gastroenterologist because Zach couldn't have his phone for long.

On day four, he was taken to the local ER because he was in such pain. An X-ray showed stool throughout his entire large intestine and they gave him an enema. He texted: *I have never been in so much pain in my life. I like the program but my stomach is not ok.* While all of this was going on, I looked at flights to NC to be with him through all of this, but by then he was already back at the treatment house.

Two days later, he was back at the hospital ER for another enema. Zach texted that they were forcing him to eat (this is an eating disorder treatment facility after all) and that it's causing him so much pain and that he's not going back. We tried to reason with him but he stopped texting. He went out and drank all night and showed up back at the treatment center at 6 am. They allowed him to stay, but he was told that he wouldn't be allowed back if it happened again. He texted us: *I'll stick it out. I'm sorry. I'm really sorry mom and dad.*

Two weeks went by and then it began all over again.

He texted that he was leaving.

> *I'm not coming home and I'm not going back there. I'm sick of all of this. The mental health, the constipation, the eating.*

I'M SICK OF IT ALL. I'm running and I don't care what happens. I quit.

Peter told him to get back to the center immediately. I pleaded with him to go back.

At this point I'm so sick of depression and anxiety and stomach problems, I don't care if I'm homeless and I die.

Then there were no more texts. I called him and he said he was going to a motel and hung up. It kept going straight to voicemail after that.

For many years, Peter had been saying that we had to prepare ourselves that we may lose Zach. We could only do the best that we could do each day, and the reality was that Zach could die. His life was a living hell most of the time and we had to accept the fact that he may take his own life, no matter how hard we tried to prevent it.

I had never accepted this. I always knew that Zach would get better, that God would heal him, and that he would someday be a counselor and help others, and he would write a book that helped others. That night as I tried in vain to go to sleep, having no idea where Zach was or what would happen, my brain had to finally accept the fact that we could lose him. I braced myself for a call from the NC police during the night. I had to mentally acknowledge this truth, still my heart would not accept it. In my heart, I always KNEW Zach would someday get better.

I got a few hours of sleep from sheer exhaustion and woke up at 6 am to a text that Zach was okay, he was at a motel. There were only a few days left of the program but he was not allowed back. He went back to get his things and got a flight home.

At this time, I had a new job hostessing at our favorite local restaurant "Poppyseed" (the BEST). I had yoga and reiki clients on some days, and worked three days at the restaurant. So I went to work that morning and put a smile on my face, exhausted from the night, but so grateful that Zach was alive.

It was at that moment that I realized how beneficial my self-care had been to my survival through all of these difficult years. My daily yoga and meditation practice truly helped get me through each day, one day at a time. This particular day I didn't have time for it because we had been on the phone all morning about Zach and I had to get to work, and I felt like a train wreck because of that. My insides felt like they were shaking all day and I couldn't catch my breath. Certainly I was depleted from the terrifying night and lack of sleep, but I knew that if I had time for my morning routine of yoga and meditation, I would have been in a better place.

This time when Zach returned from inpatient, we weren't as optimistic. He was clearly not in a good place and didn't get the help he needed at Carolina House due to all the chaos. Everything peaked; OCD, bulimia, and now his depression became worse. He had let us down, and let himself down, and that always led to deep depression.

Over the course of those years, there were arrests, countless fender benders (due to OCD), getting thrown out of bars, and even embarrassing his brothers. Even though he was an adult, we "grounded" him after every infraction because he was living with us. We would take away his car or phone or both. Some years, I think that he was grounded more days than not.

When he got into any kind of trouble, letting us down and letting himself down, he would always spiral into depression, the vicious cycle again. He would barely leave his room besides school or work.

Again we would worry about him taking his life. The cycle was mentally and emotionally exhausting for all of us. Of course this really affected his brothers by now who were always very aware of Zach's state. Additionally, we had Keith and Melissa in the family now who were affected as well. It spoke volumes of their love for Zach that they stuck around for all of it. It would get worse.

His depression worsened even more. He was going to Brylin Outpatient for group mental health meetings in addition to his psychologist and psychiatrist appointments, but there was no one that he related to and nothing seemed to be helping.

Peter took the boys to Disney World and Zach spent most of the time in the hotel room at his favorite place in the world, skipping the parks that he loved so much. This said it all. I don't think there is anything he loved more than spending a day in Disney World with his brothers. He was texting me from the room:

> The depression, anxiety, OCD, eating disorder, stomach problems. All of the treatment centers. Not to mention school and work (things normal people stress about) ... I can't keep doing this. And it's gonna continue forever. I just don't want to live anymore. And I don't think it'd be a sin to end it either.

I begged him to stay strong and I pleaded with him to go with his dad and brothers rather than sit alone in the room in this state.

> It's the same every year. I just want to die I'm sorry.

I have to mention here that Zach never talked about suicide to get attention. Back when Zach first mentioned suicidal thoughts in 2012, I had a friend who said that maybe it was for attention; that some kids were acting out and talking about suicide for attention. That was NEVER the case with Zach. He wanted to live. He was always ashamed to admit when he was feeling suicidal because he didn't want to terrify us. When he actually told us he was feeling suicidal, he was at rock bottom and had been thinking about it for awhile.

Obviously it scared me enough that he was alone in a hotel room in Disney World feeling suicidal, that I called Peter and begged him to leave the boys and go back and check on Zach. He did just that of course. All in all, it was not a fun trip for Zach and Peter.

That summer when I thought it couldn't get worse, another bomb dropped. We knew that Zach had experimented with prescription drugs in the past, but we did not know that it had escalated. And he was suicidal. As usual, he told me in a text:

Zach: *It's not just random thoughts anymore. I've been constantly thinking about how to end it, and where. And I don't know if it was before or after the pills but it feels like it's just been lingering for the past couple months and now it's non-stop.*

Me: *Do you feel unsafe right now? If you do, you need immediate help Zach. You need to call Bylin Inpatient, right? Where are you?*

Zach: *I don't feel safe. At all.*

Me: *Call Brylin RIGHT now PLEASE.*

Zach: *All of the money I've made and spent, all from the credit card and all the money I've taken from Chris, Eric and Peter have all gone to drugs. Opana, hydrocodone, valium, Xanax, more Klonopin. And the painkillers have been the most expensive and I've been doing it a lot the past couple months. And I'm really scared. I'm having mental withdrawals and I think I'm having physical withdrawals too. I've been a drug addict/a drinker for awhile and I just want to be clean. I'm sorry - they just all take the pain and the sadness and anxiety away. They do and I hate doing it but now I think I'm addicted and I'm really scared. Opana is a really strong drug and I've prob done it like 9 times in the past couple months. I don't know if this requires inpatient or brylin outpatient but I want to stop because I'm really scared. I want to do it for you and the other 3. I'm scared mom. It just helps and it numbs everything but I need help now.*

My son was now addicted to an opioid, on top of everything else he went through and I was terrified. My body went numb when I read that text. Was it because some part of my intuition knew that this would cause his death? Or was it just because opioid is a scary word for a parent? I clearly remember going to the Orchard Park High School required parent meeting and being terrified when they told us there was an opioid epidemic and heroin epidemic in Western New York, and in Orchard Park. WHAT?! Yes, kids took these painkillers for anxiety, but they are too expensive which is why they switch to heroin. There was a parent who spoke at that meeting who had lost their child to an overdose.

Every parent, as frightened as they may be, does not think this will happen to them. I was one of them. We are good parents. We give them the best of everything; a good education, sports, lessons, but most of all LOVE. This was back when Zach was just beginning all of his mental health struggles, so a part of me thought "Oh no," but I didn't really think that this would happen to us. I went home and lectured all of my boys on both opioids and heroin. They laughed at me. "MOM! We would never do heroin or pills!!"

It became apparent after appointments with his psychologist, psychiatrist and addiction counselor that Zach would need a higher level of care. He needed a 30 day rehab at the least. We gave him two choices, go to rehab or move out. We were not allowing him to do drugs at our homes and more importantly, we were concerned for his health and safety. Zach started to research places. When looking for inpatient facilities, he always wanted to find a place that treated the OCD as well, since that was always the underlying problem. Often times, facilities would claim to treat the OCD, but once he was there, Zach said that it really didn't. Rogers Behavioral in Wisconsin is highly regarded and well known for it's success rate in treating OCD and they also treated addiction, but always had a waitlist that was months long and that would not do.

I had a friend whose son had recently completed the addiction program at Huntington Creek in Pennsylvania. He loved the program and personnel and was doing really well with his recovery. Sometimes that's all we had to go on, so Zach did the intake and they had a bed available immediately. It was a six hour drive and I had to work, so Peter drove Zach there. Zach was nervous but compliant. He attempted to convince us that he could do this through outpatient in Buffalo, but we did not agree and we were not taking that chance.

I hugged him goodbye and said, "Everything will be okay. Love you."
"Bye mom. Love you too."

I prayed, "God, please heal my Zach."

Huntington was a 30 day program and did not have any sort of IOP or "step down" program after that. We did the usual counseling sessions with him on the phone and his counselor said that he was doing really well.

Summer went on without Zach. We all went out for dinner for my mom's 80th birthday. Keith and I went to his cousin's wedding in Saratoga. The bride made a speech about how grateful she was for her new husband and so grateful to be there and have this beautiful day, because she had suffered for years with her mental health and couldn't have imagined that she could be happy like this. I sat at the table and cried uncontrollably, praying that would be Zach someday. All I wanted was for him to be happy. I wasn't asking for much, just for my son to be happy at his wedding someday.

Halfway through the program, I was allowed to visit Zach and attend a counseling session. Keith drove the six hours with me and we had lunch with Zach. He looked so good, so healthy. He introduced me to his new friends, including his friend Wilson who is still in our lives. As usual, everyone loved him.

He liked the program and the counselors but at this point in his life, Zach could have been the counselor and he said as much. He had been through the 12 step program so many times, and he had been in counseling for eight years, and as every counselor always said, he was highly intelligent. I am not saying it was easy. I cannot imagine how hard it is for addicts to go through these programs, in group counseling all day, every day. As always, we told Zach how strong and courageous he was to go through these programs, but at this point Zach was almost on auto pilot; he did what he had to do to get through the month.

The biggest problem was always that instead of feeling good the way most people did after a month of sobriety, Zach felt a thousand times worse because he didn't have anything to dull the OCD symptoms.

The counselor suggested that he do a step down program at another fa-

cility, but Zach refused. He was adamant that he didn't want to miss another semester of school and be further behind. He wanted to move forward
with his life. He also did not want to miss Peter's first year of varsity football
games, both for Petes and for himself. Peter and I really felt that he should
do a step down program and if there had been one there, we would have
insisted, but the places that she suggested didn't even have a bed available
and it would be a wait. He would have to come home anyway. We also
understood how much he wanted to get on with his life. We prayed and
hoped for the best.

CHAPTER FIFTEEN

W E WERE IN A whole new phase with Zach now. As worried as we were about his mental health, his well being, and his safety, we also had difficulty trusting him now. That is a sad place to be with your son who you adore. Opioids are so highly addictive, the addict will do anything to get them. He had borrowed money from his brothers to buy pills, and nothing describes how desperate he was more than that. All he ever wanted was to make them proud and he was ashamed.

He started back at UB and working for his dad and we set up a strict schedule for him. We took away his credit card and Peter did not give him any of the money that he earned working for him; he put it in an account for him that he couldn't touch. We only gave him $3 at a time to buy a coffee. If he wanted take out food, we would call and pay over the phone. We insisted that he must attend AA meetings. If he didn't adhere to these rules and remain drug free, he could not continue to live at our homes.

This was obviously the most difficult decision we ever had to make, but we couldn't condone his drug use and it wasn't fair to the rest of the family to continue this strained and exhausting environment.

Peter began junior year of high school and it was his first year of varsity football. Our whole family was excited, especially Zach. He was so happy to be at the home opener, so proud of his brother. He asked my sister Kerry to take a picture of Zach and me and he posted it on Instagram saying:

Happy to be back.

Two weeks later, Peter called me at work to tell me that Zach was leaving. He told Peter that he couldn't live without his Klonopins and he wanted him to give him his Klonopins and he was leaving. Of course I was panicked and texted him.

> Zach: *I don't want to be homeless.. but I just don't want to deal with anxiety my whole life without Klonopin. I choose to walk out and it's my Klonopin so I get to have it. I'm leaving your house, it's mine, it's prescribed to me. Where are they?*
> *I'm leaving mom. It's my life.*

I told him not to do anything until I got there. He sent a screenshot of a text he had sent to "Gurgz", the guy who must have been supplying pills to him:

> *I'm at the wanting to die point and doing drugs is the best way I know to go out.*

I flew out of work, basically yelling out that Zach was in trouble and raced to Peter's house, calling Peter to make sure he was with Zach. If he was really leaving to go live God knows where, I needed to see him first. Maybe we should have just let him walk out and hit rock bottom alone, but the suicidal text to the drug dealer would not allow me to do that. It was another cry for help. If he wanted to leave, he would have been long gone. Later on, our family therapist strongly agreed; if Zach went to "live on the streets," we would most likely never see him again. He would probably die on the street.

After a lengthy argument, Zach reconsidered and agreed to stay and abide by our rules. He spent a couple days and nights in his room at Peter's house in a state of deep depression. One of the hardest things for me was that once Zach started doing opioids, he withdrew somewhat from me for the first time in his life. He had always confided in me, and we were always so close, but I know that he was ashamed of his drug use and didn't want to let me down, so he withdrew. He would often "hide" in his room at Peter's house, where as before, my house had always been his safe place.

A couple days later, it all came crashing down. Peter and I had been driving Zach to his psychologist appointments, AA meetings, and school because we weren't allowing him to have his car. His good friend Bethy, who'd been sober for awhile, had taken him to some AA meetings with her and had also introduced him to another guy who could give Zach rides. She always really tried to help Zach.

I always texted Bethy to make sure Zach was telling the truth. Several times I ran outside to make sure he was really being picked up for an AA meeting. This time he said he was a going to a meeting but when I checked it with Bethy, she said that neither of them had picked him up. I was at a team dinner for Peter's football team. I texted Zach.

> Me: *So are you really at a meeting? Because you're not with Bethy's friend, are you?*
>
> Zach: *Yeah you're right. I need more help mom. I've still been doing drugs and its so hard to stop. I'm gonna be home soon. I'm getting an uber back right now but I'm sorry. I need to start spending every day with dad. I'm not deliberately doing this, it's just so hard right now. I want to be drug free. I really want to but I'm scared right now. I will be home very soon. I'm scared mom. I need more help.*
>
> Me: *I'm not asking you. I'm TELLING you. Go home right now.*
>
> Zach: *I don't want to do this my whole life. I wanna finish school and help kids and I can't with this. I've been taking it out of my bank account. I'm going right now.*
>
> Me: *Do you need me to come get you? I'm at Peter's team dinner.*

Zach: *No I'm totally coherent and Uber is on way. I just need yours and dad's help. You can be on my ass. I didn't want you on my ass obv because I was still doing drugs.*

Me: *We will help you as much as you need. But I need you to go home right now. I want a picture of you at home.*

He sends me a picture of our dog Bailey as he walks into my house.

Zach: *I'm sorry. It's hard. I wish I never got into it. It's so hard to stop. I should have went to a step down.*

Me: *Yes you should have. Maybe you still can.*

Zach: *I love you guys and I love my life and I can have a good life. I don't want to be miserable and die. I don't want to die mom.*

I obviously left the team dinner early to go home to be with Zach, and I didn't let on to Petes what was going on. I remember sitting in my car doing breathing techniques to try and stay calm and centered. I felt like I was leading a double life. I taught yoga classes and did reiki on people, worked at the restaurant, cooked dinner for my boys, went to Peter's football games and looked like a normal mom doing normal mom things, but my oldest son was a drug addict.

Peter and I met with Zach to compose a plan. We took his phone away and I texted the people in his texts who had sold him drugs, begging them to leave Zach alone and begging them not to sell to him. I knew that it was a futile attempt, but I did it anyway. We called his counselor at Huntington Creek for advice. It had been too long after the 30 day rehab for a step down program to take him. He would have to do another 30 day rehab program all over again. We were back at square one.

We had two options: kick Zach out of our homes until he could figure it out and get himself clean, or send him back to another 30 day rehab inpatient. We just never could give up on him, so we were looking at a local program in Sanborn, but Peter came up with another idea. The 30 day program did the same thing over and over: keeping him drug and alcohol free plus counseling. Peter decided that he would keep Zach drug and alcohol free for 30 days at his house. He would "babysit" him at his house, at work, and at the gym for 30 days. It sounded insane, but he wanted to do it. He told me that after he did this, no matter what happened to Zach after that, he could live with himself because he had given it all he could. Whenever Peter and I discussed Zach, especially as the years got harder, he would always say, "We'll give it all we got. We'll give it all we got."

And so it began. True to his word, Peter monitored Zach 24 hours a day for 30 days. He always was a great dad. I helped with the driving to appointments and would go over and visit with him, but it was as if he was at a rehab facility because I could relax slightly because I knew he was safe.

Meanwhile, Peter was having an incredible varsity football season and Zach was at every game. On Peter's 17th birthday, it also happened to be Homecoming. He had a great game, scoring a touchdown with all of his brothers there. I took a picture of him with his brothers and it is still on his bedside table in his room. It was a pretty good birthday, to say the least.

On October 12th, Zach posted a photo of himself on Instagram in honor of World Mental Health Day,

> *I'm eternally grateful to be here and have the support of wonderful friends and family because there have certainly been very rough patches throughout the past 8 years. Been all over, met some extraordinary people and have learned so much. A special shout out to anyone who has spoken up about their struggles. It takes courage. Keep on keepin' on.*

Yes it does take courage and Zach definitely had that. He was never afraid to put it all out there and bare his problems and mistakes for the world to see. He was never afraid of being ridiculed or looking "weak," because he knew that his posts helped people to feel less alone in their struggles. I always told him how much I admired him for that. I recently read a quote that reminded me of Zach. I do not know who wrote it.

> *The beauty of you is not where you are perfect. It is where you are brave.*

CHAPTER SIXTEEN

Z ACH MADE IT though the 30 days of sobriety with Peter. Peter's football team continued to have a great season and they made it to the championship game at the Bills Stadium. We were all there of course, including Zach. Orchard Park lost the game, but what an exciting season it had been! Peter had had an incredible season, scoring a total of eight touchdowns and two interceptions. The excitement had been a welcome distraction for all of us, especially for Zach. He couldn't wait for Peter's senior year of football.

The night of the championship game, the boys were at Peter's house and he allowed Zach to go to his friend's house within walking distance. We knew the parents and he knew that they were home. Early the next morning, the friend and her dad went to Peter's house to tell him that Zach had overdosed and was taken by ambulance to Mercy Hospital. He had taken some of her Xanax on top of his prescribed Klonopin and alcohol and the parents had found him unconscious in a chair. The EMT had used Narcan on him which hadn't helped since he hadn't taken an opioid. Narcan only works on opioids.

When Peter called me, he said that Zach was okay; he was breathing on his own and was not on a ventilator. So many emotions: terror at what could have happened, anger, fear that it could happen again, relief that he was alive.

He was still in the ER when I got there. I sobbed with relief that he was conscious and would be okay. They moved him to the ICU for a couple of days to monitor him for lung damage. Peter and I would go every day and sit and stare at him. I wanted to be mad at him for what he did, but I was just so happy that he was alive. We could have lost him.

He was then transferred to a regular room for a few more days. His doctor was a young pregnant woman. She told us that Zach's heart was not the heart of a young 23 year old, but rather the heart of someone in their 40's. This was something that I had always feared. Zach had been on multiple prescribed medications for seven years, and had been bulimic on and off for five years. That alone was taxing on his heart and then for the past couple years, he had been mixing opioids and benzodiazepines (benzos) with alcohol.

Our biggest hope was that this was a huge wake up call for Zach. He was lucky to be alive and his body couldn't take much more. We asked the doctor to make sure that Zach understood the condition of his heart and she was quite direct with him. I know that she was concerned for his health and she wanted to scare him straight, but at the same time I saw judgement in her eyes; judgement of Zach and of us as parents.

It is not in my nature to be super direct. I don't like confrontation at all and quite honestly, I generally live by the "take the high road" rule when someone wrongs me. I don't know if it was my protective mama bear nature, but I felt that I had to say something to her. Before we left the hospital, I found her alone in the corridor. I asked her if this was going to be her first baby and she said no, that she had a toddler at home. I told her that when Zach was a toddler, I couldn't have imagined that this was our future. I told her that we were good parents, that my boys are my world, and that Zach was an exceptional human. I told her about Zach's debilitating OCD, anxiety disorders and depression and that was how he became addicted to pills. I told her that I hoped she would never have to experience any of this as a parent.

She was a good doctor and a kind person, but I felt that she needed to know the truth, especially for all of her future patients. The term "drug addict" has an extreme stigma to it and given the millions of people who struggle with addiction, she was lucky if it hadn't touched her personal world. I sincerely hope for her sake that it never does.

After a week, Zach was released and when I picked him up from the hospital, there was an aide taking him out in a wheelchair with me. When we got to the parking ramp and I went to get the car, the aide asked Zach why he was in the hospital. After Zach told him the story, he said, "You have a fresh start man!" I remember feeling overwhelmed with gratitude at that moment that Zach was alive. I had hope for his future and I hoped that he did too. I know that he was grateful to be alive and grateful to be going home to spend the holidays with his brothers.

It was obvious that he needed a higher level of addiction rehab for a longer amount of time. We began looking at inpatient addiction facilities once again, however the doctor had said that he had 4-6 weeks of physical recovery ahead. His lungs and his body needed time to heal and he had regular visits to his doctor. I was so thankful that he would be home for the holidays and his birthday. In retrospect, I realize that time was a gift. It would be his last holiday season with us.

I had my boys and my family for Thanksgiving dinner at my house and the Buffalo Bills game was on that night. The Bills won and my sister took a video of the boys all jumping around and yelling with excitement during the game. I love that video so much.

Zach and all of my boys are insanely dedicated Bills fans. Bills fans (commonly known as Bills Mafia) are a special breed of fans. Perhaps it's because we have never won a Super Bowl (but come so close!) or just because football in Buffalo is like a religion, but we never give up hope for our team. The standard form of hello and goodbye in Buffalo is "Go Bills!" I learned the game of football watching Bills games with my dad, another die hard fan. My boys were watching Bills games with their dad before they could even walk.

When the Bills made the playoffs in 2017 for the first time in 17 years, Zach cried, but nothing excited him more than the arrival of Josh Allen as quarterback in 2018. From day one, Zach was his number one fan. They were the same age. You probably know that now Josh Allen is one of the best quarterbacks in the NFL, but back then there were "fair weather fans" as Zach called them. He always believed in his QB, demonstrated by some of his tweets on Twitter:

> *I'm speechless with this dude's progress. Luh my QB*
>
> *Let's not hold Josh to completely unrealistic expectations now. Stay cool. He's gonna ball, no worries.*
>
> *Ride or die with my guy. Keep proving ppl wrong @joshallenqb*

He was right. He would be so proud to see his QB now.

Zach struggled with fatigue all through December but his health was slowly improving. A few days before his birthday, in the midst of us trying to figure out where he would be going for treatment in January, he sent Peter and me a text:

> *Peter got All WNY honorable mention. I said he was gonna get it with the amount of yards and TD's he had at the end of the season.*

Even with all that he was dealing with, his big brother pride prevailed over anything else.

On December 19th, we celebrated Zach's 24th birthday. He posted a picture of himself with his cake on Instagram. The post said:

> *23 was ruff. Hopefully 24 is the turnaround.*

I gave him a card and wrote: *This is your year. I just know it.*

It was his last birthday and last Christmas with him here. If only I had known, what would I have done differently? Probably nothing. We all spent time together and that's all I could ever hope for.

That Christmas morning, I took the traditional photo of the four of them. I have twenty photos on my phone and there is not one picture where they weren't being total goofballs and laughing; each one taking turns making each other laugh, doing silly gestures like when they were young boys, even at one point linking arms. Ridiculous. All I can see when I look at these photos is their pure love for each other and their unbridled joy just being together. Of course I will never delete even one of these photos. They all had their new Bills hats atop their heads and Zach was wearing his new *The Office* t-shirt.

Have I mentioned Zach's obsession with the tv show *The Office*? It's hard to even explain. It started whenever he was in a depressed state and spending many hours alone in his room, he would watch *The Office* on his laptop. It obviously made him laugh and helped get him through many hours and days. He would watch episode after episode. I have seen snippets of the show here and there, but I have never watched the whole series or even an entire episode. Zach would periodically send me a Youtube video from the show to make me laugh. He sent me the wedding scene at least three times because he knew how much it made me laugh. I love comedy and I am a big fan of Steve Carell and John Krasinski, but I could never watch the show. It has always reminded me of Zach's dark days. I still haven't been able to bring myself to watch it, but one of these days I will.

We spent the rest of the holiday season closely watching Zach and researching where he would go for inpatient. I had also told Zach about a place in New York City called the Amen Clinic that had really helped two kids that we knew. At the Amen Clinic they actually take a scan of the patient's brain (Brain Spect Imaging) to help diagnose and treat the patient. I had talked to two moms at length about how the Amen Clinic had helped their kids.

Even though we all agreed that Zach needed extensive inpatient treatment for addiction as soon as he was physically healthy, he begged to go to the Amen Clinic first. It was only a few days to do the scan and evaluation at the clinic in NYC and then he would be given a psychiatrist for follow up from home. It was $4000 but Peter agreed to pay for it and I would take him to New York. At the same time, a friend had recommended an addiction facility in Tucson, Arizona called Sierra Tucson which was highly rated. There was a bit of a wait for him to go there, so we agreed to

the Amen Clinic first. We were always searching for ways to help with the OCD which was always the underlying problem. We hoped that the Amen Clinic could help.

It was January 2020 and Zach and I left for New York City. We were required to stay for three nights because of the way the tests and scan and appointments were set up. We stayed at a hotel a few blocks from the Amen Clinic. The first morning I went with Zach to the appointment. We filled out paperwork and I waited with him until they called him back.

In the waiting room, it was just Zach and me, and another boy with his mom. He looked a little younger than Zach and it felt like he was in a cloud of darkness. His mom looked like she was on the verge of a nervous breakdown. I was all too familiar with this scene. When the boys were called in, she told me that she was at her wit's end. She didn't know how to help her son, both his dad and her fiancé had left because of him, and she didn't know what she was going to do. I was grateful that I had somehow managed to keep myself sane and balanced even through all that we had gone through with Zach. I wanted to hug her and give her some advice on how to help HERSELF; book suggestions, breathing techniques, meditation, anything, but the boys came back and I wasn't able to. I often wonder what happened to them.

Zach was free for the rest of the day, so we went off sight seeing. I always loved taking my boys to NYC and seeing it through their eyes. Ten years prior, my sister and I took the boys for a long weekend and we had the best time. We even took a photo of the boys and me on the porch of my old apartment in Hell's Kitchen. In 2013, Peter and I had taken the boys to see Christopher's CHS team in a tournament. They loved visiting NYC, but none of them wanted to live there like I had. Zach made me do every tourist thing again on this trip. He dragged me to Times Square where he asked a stranger to take a picture of us, which he posted on Instagram.

He wanted to see the Christmas tree at Rockefeller Center, where we took more photos. We had Mexican for dinner and watched the movie *Big* in our room, which Zach had never seen. I told him that the piano scene was filmed at FAO Schwarz right up the street and so the next day after his appointment, we went to FAO Schwarz. He danced on the big toy piano, smiling like a little kid. He looked happy.

I had scored some last minute tickets to *The Lion King* on Broadway. The seats were amazing. I believe angels had something to do with that. The show was phenomenal. Peter and I had taken the boys to see it in both Buffalo and Toronto when they were little, but of course Zach didn't remember it. I'll never forget the look on his face when the show ended. He said, "That was amazing!" with the biggest smile on his face. Once again, he looked like young happy Zachary at that moment.

The final morning we met with the psychiatrist to go over his scans and counseling session. It was fascinating. Every aspect of Zach was represented in the scan of his brain: OCD, depression, high intelligence, and addiction. Zach looked at me, almost with a look of "I told you." I realized at that moment that the reason he wanted the scan so badly was validation. He wanted to show all of us that he didn't make any of this up, that he didn't exaggerate. When someone has a broken bone or cancer, it's right there represented by an X-ray or scan to prove that it's there. I understood completely how Zach felt, but he knew that I ALWAYS believed him and that no one knew the depth of what he went through more than his dad and I did.

Unfortunately for us, the Amen Clinic did not help Zach and that's not completely their fault. They didn't give us all of the materials when we left; they were supposed to be emailed to Zach immediately. The suggestions for his OCD were in other countries and not feasible at this point, and the email never came. Zach called them several times, and then I called and it finally came, but he was leaving by then to go to inpatient for months. He had one appointment with the Amen Clinic psychiatrist over the phone before he left. Please know that I am not criticizing the Amen Clinic. I know that they help people; I personally know of at least two of them. It just didn't work for Zach at that time and under those circumstances.

While the NYC trip was not successful for Zach's treatment, it was a gift for me. I got to spend three whole days with my boy and it was like the old days, before the drugs. Zach knew that the scans wouldn't work if he had any drugs or alcohol in his system, so he was completely clean, completely Zach. We had so much fun.

I often wonder if Zach's soul knew what was coming, and he begged to go on this NYC trip to give me that wonderful weekend. I do know that there was some kind of fate involved and I will always be grateful for that weekend I got to spend with him. The photos that Zach wanted to take of us at Times Square and Rockefeller Center are the last two pictures that I have of the two of us. Did his soul arrange that for me? Maybe it was angels. I just know that I'm so thankful. I have a large print of the two of us in Times Square hanging in my bedroom. Behind us is the giant billboard of *The Lion King*. Of course.

A week later was my birthday and I got my usual beautiful text from Zach:

> *Happy Birthday!! You're the best mom ever and thank you for everything!*

Once again his heart shined through even though he was deep into depression again. He was in limbo, just waiting to go to Sierra Tucson. A week before he left, he posted a picture on Instagram of him and his brothers and wrote:

> *I'm a lucky SOB to have these 3 gentlemen. Just feeling a lil bit appreciative.*

CHAPTER SEVENTEEN

Zach left for Sierra Tucson on February 1st. He insisted that we not accompany him; it was his fifth time at a long term inpatient facility and he was 24 yrs old. We agreed. If there was one thing that we had learned by this point, it was that Zach had to do this on his own. Peter or I walking him to the door like we had all the times before wasn't going to make a difference. It was time for him to take complete responsibility of getting himself there and doing the work. He was the only one who could get himself clean. I hugged him goodbye and said, "Everything will be okay. Love you Zach."

"Bye mom. Love you."

I prayed, "God, please heal my Zach."

With Zach at Sierra Tucson (ST), once again we had a month of peace, knowing that he was safe and hoping that this time would be the charm. We did family counseling sessions with him by phone and as always, his counselor said that he was intelligent, kind, so grateful for his family, and very much wanting to get clean and make us all proud.

Zach liked ST a lot. He liked his counselors and per usual Zach style, had already made new friends and formed close bonds. Unfortunately as always, with all of the painkillers stripped away, the OCD became even

more severe and overwhelming without anything to numb it. After he died, one of his counselors from ST texted me:

> *There are no words that suffice in response to such a tragedy, but I am so heartbroken knowing what you are going through. I remember Zach so well and can tell you that my sessions with him brought me to tears in my supervisor's office more than once after witnessing and listening to the severity of his struggles and his desire and continued efforts to find relief from his symptoms in a way that would honor his health and the people he loved. He made an impact on me as a therapist and I will never forget him.*

The truth is, everyone who tried to help Zach felt like they failed him because nothing ever really helped the OCD. He had been in therapy for a decade. He had talked through every feeling and emotion that he'd ever had. He had done cognitive behavior therapy, and exposure and response therapy for OCD. He had been through the 12 step program for addiction three times. At the end of it all, it was the debilitating OCD that made it impossible for him to lead a happy life.

The month at Sierra Tucson went by without any problems and he was referred to a PHP (step down) called Nsight in Newport Beach, California because ST didn't have one there. Everything went downhill from there.

At PHP, they are allowed to leave the facility and have more freedom since they are slowly acclimating back to real life. A few days after he was there, we got a call that he had missed curfew and had come back drunk. The counselor said they would give him a second chance but he had to go through a 3-day detox again first at another facility. She spoke to Peter and me and told us that at this point, we had to tell Zach that he had to finish treatment or he couldn't come home. Tough love. We had talked about this before Zach left Buffalo, but didn't know if we could really tell Zach that he couldn't come home if he left treatment. We prayed that we wouldn't have to find out.

We all had a phone session with Zach and told him that if he left treatment again and he was kicked out of the center, he could not come home. The counselor assured us that this was the only thing left to do to help him and maybe he had to hit rock bottom. (In my mind I thought, "Really? Hadn't he already hit rock bottom several times before?!")

We had certainly heard this in drug counseling before, although all of his previous counselors did not agree this would be the best route for Zach. Yet here we were. Zach understood. I was terrified.

A few days later, we got the call that he was gone and he had stolen someone's prescription meds. He knew he couldn't come home if he didn't go back. I couldn't breathe. I texted him:

Me: *Please stay strong. Don't give up.*

Zach: *I already am like 10 drinks in. I'm sorry mom. Thank you for the support and for everything throughout the years. I love you. I don't really know what I'll do out here. I'm sorry I just had to go out and drink.*

Me: *Zach I love you more than you will ever know (until you have a child of your own.. then you'll know). You need to get yourself sober. You know you do. You always have our support. Go back to Nsight and hopefully they will take you back. Talk to your counselors and friends. You need help. Please keep fighting.*

Zach: *I love you mom. I'm sorry. I don't wanna feel like this but I can't help it. I hope I can see you soon. Thank you for everything. I already did but please tell Christopher Eric and Peter I love them more than anything. I can't stop crying mom. Thank you for everything.*

Me: *You're gonna be okay! I know you are. You always have a family. Go back to Nsight and fight to live . I KNOW YOU CAN DO IT. I love you.*

And that was it. There was no more contact after that. I felt like the worst mom in the world. We had had addiction counselors tell us in the past to give him the ultimatum of treatment or move out. We had given him that ultimatum several times and he had always chose treatment. My heart was in my throat.

Then the texts started coming from our boys. Of course Zach had texted them and they were irate. We tried to explain that this was the only way Zach would get clean, but they wouldn't hear of it. They also had not been through all of the addiction counseling that we had. Christopher said that he was driving to L.A. to get Zach. Not only was he on the streets of L.A., but Covid 19 had just hit our country hard and everything was on lock down. I wanted Zach home too.

The next day we got a call from Nsight that he was back. Thank God. He had gone to the streets of L.A. and traded his jacket that I had bought him for Christmas for drugs. Then he had stayed at a friend's apartment; he knew her from Buffalo. Nsight was allowing him back, but he had to go through the 3-day detox again. (All of this kept adding to the bill that Peter got.) It was like being on a terrible roller coaster ride.

He then had a new therapist that agreed that from there, Zach should transfer to an inpatient facility that also specialized in OCD treatment. They were looking at one in Houston, but because of Covid, it was online only. The waitlist for Mclean OCD Institute in Boston was six months and the wait for Rogers Behavioral Hospital in Wisconsin was four months.

Zach texted me:

> *The new therapist reads my mind. People can do AA all they want to stay sober, but when I do the program, my OCD gets worse, like it was here. This is the reason I use. It's not the opposite. If I didn't have OCD or anxiety or any mental health issues, I wouldn't have drinking or drug problems. I'm not doing this purposely. I just want to quiet my mind. I think I need a higher level of care. I feel like such a burden to everyone in the family. I sound like a broken record but I*

don't mean to drink or use drugs to suppress my emotions, it just takes away the pain. I just feel like I'm a burden on our family and on yours and dad's relationships. I want to stop badly because now I know how it affects everyone in my life.

Me: *It does affect everyone Zach but you're NOT a burden. You're a blessing. Remember that.*

Because of the long waitlists for OCD inpatient facilities, the plan was for Zach to go to Sierra by the Sea in California, basically starting the 30 day rehab all over again, however it all fell apart because of Covid. They were now understaffed and unable to provide the full program, so Zach wasn't able to go there. The only choice at this point was for him to come home.

He came home on April 3rd and we were never so happy to see him. He posted on Twitter when he got home:

My life will suffice, no matter how short or long, as long as I made people happy.

More foreshadowing?

Zach got home just in time for us to say goodbye to our beloved Bailey, our golden retriever of twelve years. She had cancer and had surgery a couple months before, but it hadn't helped. She was suffering and could barely move so we had to put her down. She was a member of our family. My boys literally grew up with her.

Our Bailey had a beautiful life. She had four brothers who were always throwing a ball around and she had her own swimming pool. She was a swimming nut. She dug a hole under the pool fence so she could slide in and swim all day long. She had crazy energy (I'm sure that living with four boys and all of their crazy energy contributed to that), but she was the sweetest dog ever. We called her Bae. She was a big pile of love.

Covid had hit New York state as well and everything was completely shut down. The vet clinic was open, but in order to put a pet down, you could only drop them off and you weren't allowed to stay with them. There was no way I was going to have my girl go through that alone. I was staying with her to the end. My friend suggested a vet who comes to your house to put your pet down and as odd as that sounds, it was perfect.

When she was a young dog at our old house, Bailey always slept at the top of the stairs between all of our rooms like a guard, but now she couldn't climb stairs. When I came downstairs on her last morning, she was laying in a pool of sunlight. It was as if angels were already surrounding her.

We all gathered around her in the family room: my boys, Peter, my sister Kerry, Keith and me. She could see everyone that she loved most in the world and she wasn't at all scared. Her head was in my lap. It was sad and beautiful at the same time. I now believe that Bailey left at that exact time so that she could be there for Zach when he crossed over.

This was a very difficult way for all of us to begin the Covid months and I worried about Zach because he was already not in a good place. Zach's love of animals ran so deep and this was his girl. He took it really hard, as we all did.

As for me, I am a dog lover to say the least. We had a family dog when I was growing up (Buttons), but I have owned my own dog my entire adult life. I feel like all of my dogs were soulmates of mine. My first dog was a Siberian Husky named Shetan who Peter bought me for my 21st birthday. She lived with me at two different apartments, my parents' house, Peter's parents' house, and finally at our house. We had her for nine years before Zach was even born so she was like our first kid. We had to put her down when I was pregnant with Eric and we were so devastated, we waited eight years before getting another dog.

Bailey came at the time of our divorce, but she usually went where the boys were so she spent a lot of time at Peter's house and he adored her. After we lost Bailey, I absolutely knew that I would get another dog, but I needed some time to mourn my girl. The house was sad and quiet without her. Keith and I had adopted a cat named Kobe in 2014 and I loved him, but there was a void without Bailey. Kobe missed her too.

Losing Bailey was not a good start to Zach's re entry into "normal" life and to make matters worse, the Covid lockdown had just begun. Gyms, restaurants, schools, everything was shut down and there was nowhere to go. This plus the general Covid based fears that affected most humans, affected a kid who had already been dealing with severe OCD, depression and addiction and had just come out of two months of rehab even more so.

Covid also really affected seniors in high school and college that year. Normal celebrations and ceremonies were nonexistent for most seniors. Christopher was hit hard by this. He was graduating from Mercyhurst University with a BA in business marketing. He had lived with his college friends for years and they were like family to him. Instead of having their last couple months together and graduating together, they had a day's notice to pack up and move out for good.

He didn't even get so much as a virtual graduation ceremony after four years of hard work and a college degree. It was so disappointing for me as well, to not get to see my son graduate from college. I could tell that Christopher was having a hard time as well, having to abruptly leave school and his busy life to be sitting at home all the time.

A few months later when restaurants opened up, we had a graduation dinner for him with our parents and sisters. It was wonderful and I realize now that one of the best things about it was that my sister Kerry took a bunch of photos that day. In particular, there is a photo of Peter and the boys with our dads, and also a photo of the boys and me. That would be the last time that Peter and I would get a photo with all four of our sons. There is also a photo of my four boys. It's the last photo of them together. I am so grateful to have these photographs.

As happy and proud as Zach was of Christopher, Peter and I knew that it was difficult for him to see Christopher and his friends graduating from college while he was still plugging along. We always told him that he was on his own timeline and not to compare himself to others, especially since he had taken time off to do so much difficult work on himself in treatment. It was so impressive to me that he always chose to go back to UB and keep working towards his degree. That summer he did online classes due to Covid. He and his brothers also worked for their dad all summer which helped keep them somewhat busy.

Even with the difficult circumstances, Zach stayed clean in the beginning. He started seeing a new psychologist, Dr. Chris Fitzgerald, who specialized in OCD treatment. He was actually Peter's step brother's best friend. Zach really liked him and trusted him, and he said that he was the first psychologist or therapist to really help with his OCD since his psychologist at the Children's Psychiatric Clinic two years before.

Every now and then, Chris would have Peter and I come in with Zach for a session to keep us in the loop. He seemed familiar to me, but I couldn't place it. Soon after, Zach told us that he realized that Chris had been his counselor at a summer camp that he went to when he was young. He was his favorite counselor. So ironic, but it didn't surprise me at all. It's funny how people are placed in our lives.

Chris brought up Rogers Behavioral again and proposed that it be a final resort for Zach. Zach, as always, did not want to go away; he wanted to stay on track at UB and continue working with Chris. He said that he helped him. That was the plan for now.

CHAPTER EIGHTEEN

In May of 2020, Zach's friend Lilly that he had met at Sierra Tucson came to visit from New Jersey. Because we have so many Lily's, I call her Lilly B. They had a fun couple of days as he showed her around WNY and then because her dad had driven her from New Jersey and was coming back to pick her up, Zach drove her halfway. On his drive back, he drank. By the time he was an hour from home, he was speeding and was pulled over by a police officer, arrested, and given a DWI. Peter went to pick him up from the police station and the arresting officer told Peter that "He was such a nice young man, I didn't want to arrest him." I can't make this stuff up. So typical Zach. Everyone loved him, even when he had done something so dumb and dangerous.

We were obviously hugely disappointed and concerned that Zach had been drinking and driving. We were back on the roller coaster. He was legally allowed to drive, but we grounded him for what felt like the hundredth time. We weren't allowing him to drive and he could only go to work and back. He had to go to court for the DWI and was put on a six month probation where he would be tested periodically for drugs and alcohol. If he failed the test, he would go to jail.

It was difficult for us to be optimistic. Six months seemed like an eternity and Zach's track record wasn't good. I had a perpetual stomach pain.

I couldn't imagine my intelligent, kind, compassionate son, who had so much to offer this world, going to prison and yet it was a reality. Peter had a friend who was familiar with life with an addict and he had told him that there were only three outcomes for an addict: sobriety, jail, or death. Zach would have to choose sobriety sooner than later or he would most likely be going to prison.

Even with all that had happened, Zach had hope. He wrote on Twitter:

> *I'm just glad I'm feeling like myself again. Each day is a chance to lift yourself a little higher. Long and difficult road ahead but there are too many important people and things in my life to give up on myself yet again. Always... Yepp.*

It gave me hope that he had hope.

Jillian asked me to make some yoga videos for her channel and she also coerced me into finally creating a website for my business. I am completely technically challenged. I tried doing a "build your own site" and it was too stressful for me, especially with all that was going on. I asked Zach to help me because he was good at all of that. He was so endearingly patient with me while I had a total meltdown. He was so kind and uncomplaining and never judged my lack of technical knowledge. It was ironic... the roles had reversed from the days when I helped him with his homework. I experienced firsthand why he would be an amazing teacher or counselor for kids.

I would be remiss if I didn't mention how passionate Zach was about social injustice. That May, George Floyd had been killed by a police officer, which spurred protests all over the United States. Americans were outraged and saddened (including me), but Zach seemed to feel it on a whole other level. He was such a sensitive soul (hence all the anxiety) and such an empath, that he felt other people's pain so deeply. There was a small protest in Orchard Park and Zach pulled over and joined in. We later found his hand made sign in his car. On August 26th, he tweeted:

> *It shouldn't be difficult, it really shouldn't. Stop unjustly killing black men, women and children.*

He had no tolerance for mistreatment of any humans or animals.

Keith and I did our annual visit to Saratoga and it was difficult for me because I felt like Zach was not good and not saying anything about it. I was texting with him from there and he texted:

> *Have fun mom. I've just been pretty down and a little worried. But I think I've got it.*

The probation officers still hadn't contacted him because of Covid delays. I texted back:

> *I understand. Just remember 'This too shall pass.' I know you've got this. Love you.*

By end of August, just as UB was starting, I sensed that Zach was worse. I texted:

> *Zach I feel like you're struggling and not saying anything. I am here for you. Nothing is more important to me than your well being. If you need help, please reach out. I know you want to go to UB, but you can get help locally. Please talk to me when you need to.*

> Zach: *Maybe I should go somewhere.*

> Me: *Like a rehab?*

> Zach: *No. Somewhere like Rogers. There have been bad thoughts last night and today.*

> (Meaning suicidal thoughts.)

> Me: *Do you need to go to Brylin?*

> Zach: *I don't think so.*

He tried to keep going and continued going to work and school. I sent him a meme that said:

> *One day you will tell your story of how you overcame what you went through and it will be someone else's survival guide.*

I truly believed that with all my heart.

A week later he texted:

> *I'm not feeling that great. I was really depressed today and left Christopher at the office and just parked somewhere and slept in my car. I don't think dad knows that. It wasn't just depression. I was thinking about the future and had no excitement or happiness or motivation. I realistically almost was just gonna drive away somewhere, I don't even know where. So I just parked and slept. I just don't know if I can even function as a normal human being to be honest. I don't see myself being able to have a real job or finish school or live a life. I just see myself in and out of treatment centers for the rest of my life.*

I talked him off of the ledge, reminding him that he always has ebbs and flows, ups and downs. His psychologists had always reminded him of that, but we also always told him to let us know if he needed a higher level of care. There was nothing worse than hearing my son say that he didn't think he would ever have a happy life. Jillian had previously told me that whenever Zach was in a very bad place and I felt myself consumed with worry and fear, that I should close my eyes and picture him happy. She said that worry and fear obviously did nothing to help him, that I should focus on raising my vibration and that WILL help him. So whenever I meditated, I would picture Zach holding his newborn baby, with the biggest smile on his face, happy. So happy. I did that so many times that I felt that it was real, that I was seeing the future.

In September, the probation officers came to my house looking for Zach. After their visit Zach said they were very nice. Then he told us that he had been doing Opana again. As usual, he texted me:

> *I need to go somewhere. Inpatient.*

He admitted that he had done Opana six times since he found out he was on probation three months ago. We asked him how that could be since we hadn't allowed him to have any cash or credit card. He had written down numbers of our credit cards and used a cash app. (I didn't even know what that was.) I had a debit card which is where my Covid unemployment was deposited to when the restaurant was closed and Zach had taken over $1000 from it. Opana is extremely expensive. It is also so highly addictive, it was taken off the market in 2017 and is only available for purchase on the street.

We were devastated to say the least. Once again we had to make a choice: kick Zach out of our homes for stealing money and doing drugs, or help him. It was an easy choice for Peter and me. We had to follow our gut instinct and continue to help him. His psychologist agreed. He was severely depressed and at times, suicidal. My friend Lisa's daughter reached out to me one night that she was really concerned about a snapchat that Zach had posted. He told us that he was okay, but he was clearly suicidal at times. He didn't feel that he needed to go to Brylin, but he did the intake for two out of state inpatient rehab facilities. Because we were still mid Covid, the wait was even longer than usual.

While we waited for him to get in and for a bed to become available, we guarded him twenty-four hours a day. We guarded him to keep him from being able to get drugs or alcohol, and we guarded him from being able to take his life. Of course that isn't really possible, but we tried. He spent most of the month of September in his room in the dark, watching *The Office* on his phone.

I always tried to get him off social media. To me, social media has some benefits, but the negative far outweighs the positive. It is such a difficult world for the young adults to navigate since the arrival of social media. To see all of your "friends" happy, perfect, filtered posts is difficult for all of us who are going through tough times, but for a young person like Zach who felt that he would never finish college, or have a happy relationship, or just live a "normal" life, it was downright detrimental.

As we waited the two agonizing weeks for Zach to be accepted at one of the inpatient facilities, we found out that he had finally gotten into Rogers after being on the waitlist for months. This seemed like a dream come true.

Not only was Rogers well known for their treatment of OCD, they also had a detox and addiction program, so he would be spending a long time there and getting what we hoped would be the OCD treatment that he so desperately needed.

Peter and Zach and I had an appointment scheduled with Chris, his psychologist, for October 1st to work out all of the details of the plan. In the meantime, in the background, life went on. Christopher had decided to move to Tampa, Florida and look for a job down there. That week, he packed up his car and left. I was excited for him to begin a new chapter, but so sad to see him pull out of my driveway with all of his belongings in his car. I also had tremendous guilt that I didn't drive with him, but with Zach's condition, I didn't feel that I could leave.

The weekend before the appointment for Zach was Keith's 50th birthday and I hosted a birthday dinner with our friends. Three days later was my Peter's 18th birthday. He had started his senior year of high school during Covid, so he only went to school with half of the kids he knew, and his senior football season was indefinitely postponed. We planned on going out for a birthday dinner, but his birthday fell on a Monday so in the meantime, we just had birthday cake with the family. Our family was all at my house and Zach, who had been in bed all day, came downstairs to sing happy birthday but disappeared back to his room immediately afterwards.

The next day was Tuesday and the boys were sleeping at their dad's house because he had asked to switch Tuesday for Wednesday that week because he had plans. (Our boys always followed the schedule even when they were adults with cars.) Since we weren't allowing Zach to have his car, Peter came to pick Zach up and I was just getting back from a walk when they were pulling out. Peter stopped and rolled the window down and jokingly said, "Say goodbye to your mommy." Zach smiled at me and said, "Bye mom."

I said, "Bye Zach. See you tomorrow. Love you!"

It was the last time I saw him conscious. Maybe my soul knew that, because I took a snapshot in my head of Zach smiling at me through the open window. I carry that snapshot in my heart.

The next night the boys came to my house, but Zach asked to stay in his room at Peter's house. Peter and Eric and I were switching mattresses upstairs to give Peter the newer mattress that Christopher was now not using. We were preoccupied when Eric got a text from Zach asking if one of us could pick him up and bring him to my house. By the time Eric saw the text and told Zach that I would come get him, Zach said, *Never mind*. He stayed at Peter's house. I asked Zach if he was sure and he said yes. I texted him: *Nite Zach. Love you.* It was the last text that he received.

CHAPTER NINETEEN

AT 1:30 AM I WOKE up suddenly and my phone was bright; someone was calling. I always keep my phone on "do not disturb" at night so I'm not awakened by late night texts. I have it on a setting that if anyone on my "favorites" list (including all of my sons) calls, their call will come through. Peter's fiancé Melissa was not yet on that list. That is how I know divine guidance took place. I never would have seen Melissa's call had I not woken up at that exact moment and I feel certain that it was my angels who woke me up. Melissa said simply, "Can you come here right away," but it was the near hysteria in her voice that made my blood run cold. I said, "What's wrong?" and she responded, "Just come here!"

I barely remember grabbing a sweater and shoes. Keith asked me if I wanted him to come with me and I yelled out, "Stay with Eric and Peter!" as I ran down the stairs. The drive to Peter's house is about six minutes but I think I made it in three minutes. There was no one on the road. While I was speeding, I was chanting "Please angels send light to Zach. Please angels send light to Zach."

The scene I pulled up to was like a scene from a movie, a tragedy. There were more ambulances, EMTs, and police cars than I could count, their lights flashing in the dark in complete silence. I pulled onto someone's lawn and ran towards Peter's house. At that point, I felt like I wasn't in my body anymore; as if I was watching the scene from above, but still in it. I now understand how PTSD (post-traumatic stress disorder) works. When a situation is too horrific for a person to absorb, our mind (and I believe our soul) detaches us from it, because we simply wouldn't be able to handle it. Then slowly over time, our mind brings us back to the memories of it and we allow ourselves to feel it deeper and deeper each time. That is not a medical definition; that is completely my own experience.

I felt like I watched myself run in through the side door to the front living room, where the scene that unfolded was every parent's worst nightmare. Zach was laying on the floor, surrounded by medics who were administering CPR. I saw Peter. I saw Melissa. Their faces reflected the horror that I felt. I watched myself run through all of the people onto my knees next to Zach. I put my hands on his legs, giving him reiki and praying. After a minute, I heard someone yell, "Get her out of there!" and realized that he was talking about me. I reluctantly took my hands off of Zach and stepped back.

After about twenty minutes, which felt like two hours, they got a heartbeat. They put him on a gurney and into the ambulance. I asked if Peter and I could ride in the ambulance with him but they said no, we could follow them to Mercy Hospital. Peter and I followed the ambulance. At that point, I felt like I was back in my body and I could breathe fully again. He was going to be okay.

Peter told me that he had fallen asleep on the couch and woke up and saw Zach in the other room on the floor, unconscious. He and Melissa gave him CPR but Zach did not have a heartbeat. He said that Zach had looked peaceful.

I realized that I had Zach's phone in my hand and didn't remember taking it. As I read his texts, I saw that his last conversation was with his ex-girlfriend Lily, and that his last text was from me, *Nite Zach. Love you.* I saw that a girl he knew had brought Opana to Peter's house. I texted her, explaining what had happened and asked her exactly what she had brought him, but she did not respond. She was probably scared. I do not blame her in any way. I know that she didn't want this to happen.

When Peter and I got to the ER, they put us in a little exam room and a doctor came right in. We all had masks on because of Covid procedure and I could see it all in his eyes. He said, "Your son basically died in the ambulance." They were able to get a heartbeat eventually, but it was a long time that he wasn't getting any oxygen to his brain and now in the ER, his heart had stopped again. I think I shrieked, "BUT YOU'LL KEEP TRYING! RIGHT?!" The shrill voice that came out of me didn't even sound like mine. He nodded and said yes but he didn't look hopeful.

I have no idea how long it was before he came back and said that Zach had a heartbeat, but reminded us that he had gone a long time without oxygen to his brain and didn't know how much brain function he would have. He brought us into the ER operating room to see Zach. For the rest of my life, I will never forget the looks of pity on the faces of the medical staff. They looked at us as if he was already dead, but all we cared about was that he was still alive. He was on a ventilator, but he was alive. I was hopeful. I put my hand on his head and would have stayed there, but they were taking him up to the ICU. We kissed him and told him we loved him.

Then someone took us up to the ICU waiting room where we had sat a year ago when he had overdosed. Back then, the room had been filled with people. Now with Covid restrictions, people weren't even allowed in the waiting room. Peter and I were the only ones in there and we were left there all night with no idea what was going on.

I texted my sister. I texted Dr. Chris and told him that we would not be at the appointment for Zach which was scheduled for that morning. I didn't text our boys because I was not telling them what happened in a text. I told Keith that as soon as we heard from the doctor, I would FaceTime him and he could give Eric and Peter the phone so I could tell them. It was pointless for them to come to the hospital now since they wouldn't be allowed upstairs with us. We wouldn't tell Christopher in Tampa until we knew more. We were sitting uncomfortably upright in chairs and would nod off occasionally, but for the most part we were up all night. I sent distance reiki to Zach as much as I could before I would nod off.

It was morning before the doctor came to get us. He brought us into a conference room and apologized for leaving us there all night, but he said that Zach's heart had stopped three more times during the night and they were concerned that he had gone too long without oxygen and that he didn't have brain function. They would be testing his brain function later in the day. He said the prognosis wasn't good. We just stared at him in silence, and in tears. We were in shock. We really thought that he had pulled through and would somehow be okay. I felt like the world was spinning around me and I was motionless... and powerless. It was one of the worst moments of my life. At the same time, I felt sorry for him, having to give us this horrific news.

We were allowed to see Zach. I just wanted to touch him, to touch his hair and hold his hand. We then had to FaceTime Eric and Peter, who were still asleep, to tell them what had happened. Keith was going to bring them to the hospital. We called Christopher in Tampa to tell him that his big brother was in a coma and that he had to get on the next flight home and come to the hospital. It hurts my heart to think of my 22 year old boy getting on a plane by himself, knowing that his brother was in a coma and not knowing if he would live. He said it was the only time in his life that he couldn't fall asleep on a plane.

Eric and Peter got there and it was heartbreaking to see their faces when they saw Zach, trying to fight back the tears in their eyes, trying to be strong. Again because of Covid restrictions, we were only allowed to have two people in his room so Peter took the boys down to the lobby and I stayed with Zach all day while people rotated coming up to see him. By that time, our sisters and Peter's dad and cousins were there. My parents were not able to come because they both were in such poor health. Nobody was even allowed in the hospital main lobby because of Covid, so our entire family stayed in the vestibule with one seat.

I just sat with Zach all day, holding his hand and touching his hair. I gave him reiki. I talked to him. I told him that he was going to be okay. I begged him to stay.

I prayed, "GOD, PLEASE HEAL MY ZACH!"

I begged God to take me instead. "Please take me instead of him! He's better than me. Take me. Take me."

I pleaded with God to inflict anything else on me … "Give me cancer, cut off my arm, cut off my leg, just please don't take my son! I can handle anything but that."

And then I stopped. I stopped begging because if there is one thing that I knew, one of my life lessons that I've learned, is that that's not how it works. We don't get to barter. This was Zach's journey and I had no control over it. Just as I had no control over his life before that. We cannot control what happens to the ones we love. The phrase "It's God's Will" had never been so clear to me.

As I sat, I had Zach's phone and all day long he was getting messages from friends. He had posted an Instagram story the night before, talking about his struggles and that he was going away to an inpatient again and this time he was going to get better. I cannot even begin to count how many people messaged him that they were proud of him, that they were rooting for him, that they loved him. I wish I could thank every one of them for their supportive messages, even though my Zach never saw them because he was in a coma.

Peter and I had been holding out for a miracle because miracles happen every day, but by afternoon the doctors tested his brain function and it was not good. Then his kidneys were failing so we had to make the decision to put him on dialysis. I could tell that the doctor thought it was futile at this point, but it was our choice and Peter and I made the decision to do everything we could. As a last resort, they were going to lower his body temperature to see if that helped his brain function and they would test him again in the morning for the last time.

It was at that time that I stopped putting my energy into begging Zach to stay and begging God for a miracle. Instead, I put my energy into sending

Zach light and telling him that if it was his time and he had to go, it was okay and I wouldn't leave his side. I would always be his mom and I would love him forever.

The day seemed like an eternity while I sat with Zach and our family and friends took turns coming up to see him. At one point I had fallen asleep on Zach, holding his hand and I woke up to see Francine staring at me in horror. I cannot imagine what that looked like for her, seeing our beautiful boy on a ventilator and me huddled over him, as if I was trying to keep him here.

Christopher arrived in Buffalo and his girlfriend McKenzie picked him up and brought him straight to the hospital. For the rest of this life, I will never be able to wipe from my memory the looks on my three sons' faces as they hovered around their big brother, their best friend, realizing that they were probably going to lose him. I felt responsible, like I had let all of them down.

When evening came, the nurse informed us that because of Covid restriction, we would not be able to stay all night with Zach. We had to leave. I begged and pleaded with the nurse to just let me stay with him, but they wouldn't allow it. I was terrified that he would die alone overnight, without me there. And so we all went home.

I don't remember if we ate. I don't remember anything except that I had never been so tired in my life and I actually fell asleep for a few hours out of pure exhaustion. The plan was for Peter to pick me up early the next morning because we had to meet with the medical team at 8:00 am when they would test his brain function for the last time. The boys and the rest of our family would follow since they weren't allowed upstairs with us and would have to stay in the vestibule again.

CHAPTER TWENTY

I WOKE UP TO what I already knew would be the worst day of my life. Every part of my intuition, every cell in my body, and the deepest part of my soul knew that Zach was going to die. I already knew what the brain function test would tell us. I wasn't being negative. I just knew. For so many years, I had complete optimism and eternal hope that Zach would someday be okay, but now I knew that wasn't going to happen.

Peter picked me up on a cold and rainy Friday morning. He knew too. We were both strangely calm, even though we knew that we were going to see our Zach for the last time. It was so surreal driving through our town while people were going about their normal day and we were on our way to say goodbye to our son.

I was so grateful that Zach had made it though the night. I went back to my position sitting next to him, holding his hand. He was so cold. I told him that it was okay to go. I thanked him for fighting for so long, not just for the past couple days, but for so many years. The medical team assembled in his room. There were so many of them. It was overwhelming on so many levels. I had to keep reminding myself to breathe, just breathe. I couldn't even look as they performed the test, poking and prodding him. It didn't take long.

The head doctor took us aside. He said that Zach did not have any brain function. Even though I knew that was coming, I felt as if my legs were giving way beneath me. I wasn't sure how I was still standing. He was very kind. He said that he had a 24 year old son as well. (In my head, I was thinking, "Yes, but yours is alive.") He asked us to sign a DNR. His exact words were, "Please don't make me pound on this boy's chest again."

He didn't have to convince us. While we had held onto hope the first day, we would not allow Zach to stay in this state. I personally would have taken care of him for the rest of my life, but we knew that we couldn't let him live brain dead while his body slowly deteriorated. Zach would not have wanted that. The doctor hugged us both. It was like a nightmare that wouldn't end and we couldn't wake up from. I can only imagine how grateful that doctor was to go home and hug his 24 year old son that day.

I felt like I was watching from outside my body again. Once again, my brain (or my soul?) knew how much I could handle and now we had to go downstairs to tell our sons that Zach was going to die today. Somehow my body went through the motions, but the emotion, the pure terror of what was happening was buried, to reappear at a later time. They all knew by our faces as we approached them.

We brought the boys up to see Zach. I could barely look at their faces. I kept hugging them, but the pain on their faces will always haunt me. The only pain as great as losing my Zach was the pain of knowing that my boys were losing their big brother. We huddled around him. I just kept holding his hand and touching his face, for as long as I could.

We talked about donating Zach's organs. It's what he always wanted. We met with the woman who handled organ donation and she scheduled a surgery at 4:00 that day when they would take him off the ventilator and remove his liver to be given to someone that day. I said that I would only agree to it if I could be in the surgery room when they took him off the ventilator. I had promised Zach that I would be there with him when he crossed over. They agreed to it.

Zach's nurse who was with us for the two days was so kind to us. She was a mother too. There were only supposed to be two at a time in his room but under the circumstances, she allowed all five of us to stay with Zach. Another thing I will be eternally grateful for. And so we waited.

I know that by this time, our entire community was praying for Zach and for us. He was so very loved. I can tell you that we absolutely felt those prayers. It's hard to even explain, but it was as if there was a loving energy holding us up. The light that was being sent to us from so many people (and so many angels) was helping us get through every awful moment. I believe that those prayers helped get us through the days that would follow as well. At one point, as I looked out of Zach's hospital room window, I saw a double rainbow. I took it as a sign that Zach would be lovingly guided to the other side.

Peter went downstairs to the vestibule to tell the rest of our family what was happening with the organ donation surgery. While he was gone, Zach's heartbeat flatlined. Christopher and Eric and Peter and I were frozen. Zach's nurse came running in and said, "He decided. He wasn't waiting. He's gone."

I was in shock. What do you mean he's gone?! We were supposed to go to surgery. I was going to be able to say goodbye and kiss his head one last time. I think because I was in such shock, I just grabbed his head, saying over and over "NO!!!! Please don't go Zachy. Please please please. Please Zachy don't go." I was crying hysterically. And then I remembered that my boys were there and I pulled it together for them, even though it was the worst moment of my life.

He was still breathing because he was on a ventilator, even though he was gone. The nurse removed the ventilator and I watched my baby take his last breath. While my heart felt like it had physically shattered at that moment, I was also grateful that I was there when my beautiful boy took his first breath, and I was there when he took his last breath. I had promised him that I would be with him when he crossed over, and I was. I felt calmness wash over me. He looked beautiful, peaceful. His eyes were open a little bit and he looked like he was smiling. I am sure that he was smiling at Little Grandma and Nolan and Bailey.

Peter wasn't there. I told the boys to text him and tell him to come up immediately. The second worst moment of my life was telling Peter that Zach was gone. The sheer pain on his face was a mirror to my own pain. He too couldn't believe he was gone and wasn't prepared. My poor boys. I wish they didn't have to see each of their parents go through that, but I am grateful they were able to say goodbye to their brother. We will never know why Zach chose to leave when Peter wasn't there, and his mom had done the same. Perhaps they both just didn't want to put him through that.

He died at 11:50 am on October 2nd. Our boy was gone. As calm as I felt, it was surreal. It could not be real. This wasn't what life was supposed to be. This must be a nightmare that I would wake up from. I just knew that I never wanted to leave that room. I never wanted to leave him. Somehow, as long as I was with him, he was still here.

His nurse made a handprint mold and took locks from his hair for me. She let us have our whole family up to say goodbye. Peter's cousin's priest came in to do last rites. I told him that we would only do this as long as the words judgement or hell were not used, because I don't believe in that. It was actually really beautiful. We all held hands, forming a circle with me holding one of Zach's hands and our cousin holding his other hand. It felt like angels were in the room. I could feel Zach still with us. Perhaps he was transitioning over. I clearly heard Peter's mom say, "I've got him." Yes. I knew that she did. They were reunited. It felt peaceful.

Everyone left the room except for Peter and the boys and me. It was time to say goodbye. This I did not handle well. This was the moment I had dreaded and now that the time came, I didn't really know how I was going to physically walk out of that room, away from Zach. We said goodbye again. I told him I loved him and thanked him for being the best son a mom could hope for. I made a promise to Zach that day that I would never let his name be forgotten. I would keep his memory alive and we would do great things in his name. "I love you Zach. I love you so much Zach-a-doo."

Finally, Peter was the one to have the strength to say, "Okay it's time to go."

I couldn't let go of Zach. I just kept touching his hair and kissing him on the head. When my boys were little, I always said hello or goodbye or goodnight by kissing the top of their head. As Zach got older and was taller than me, he would drop his head so that I could still kiss the top of his head. I could not accept that this was the last time that I could kiss the top of his head. The next time I saw him, he would be in a coffin and it wouldn't even be him. I JUST COULDN'T LEAVE HIM.

I heard Peter say, "Christopher, get your mom." I let Christopher pull me away from Zach because I knew I couldn't do it. I don't know how I walked out. I don't remember my legs even walking. I think Christopher was holding me up as I walked. I don't remember how we even got downstairs.

I cannot imagine what the five of us must have looked like, walking towards our family in the vestibule; the five of us without Zach. My sister told me that I looked like a shadow of myself walking towards her, and that moment haunts her. I couldn't believe I was getting into a car in the exact spot outside Mercy Hospital that we had put Zach into the car after he was born. I was leaving my baby, my first born son, my Zach-a-doo in the very hospital he was born in. As we drove away, it felt to me like darkness set in. Just DARKNESS. As if the world had gone dark.

PART 3

Finding Light Through the Darkness

"The wound is where the light comes in"
- Rumi

CHAPTER TWENTY ONE

GRIEF. I READ somewhere: "Grief never ends... but it changes. It's a passage, not a place to stay. Grief is not a sign of weakness, nor a lack of faith... It is the price of love."

It certainly is the price of love. After Zach died, the word "grief" didn't seem like an adequate word to describe what I was going through. I had known grief before when Peter's mom died, when my grandparents died, when my dogs died. That grief could not be compared to this dark emptiness I had entered into. I always say that there is no word in the English language to describe the pain of losing a child. Heartbreaking, tragic, devastating, and even horrific are overused words that don't come close to describing the pain. My heart felt like it was shattered into a million pieces. I felt as though a piece of my soul was missing.

The day that Zach died, I texted my Jillian:

He's gone.

Jillian texted:

Sending you all the light I have in my heart. He is NOT gone. It's an opportunity for a new beginning. He is in your soul group and will stay there with all of you. He is right beside you and will stay there always. Zach wants me to tell you that all you ever wanted was for him to feel happy and at peace. He feels that now. He knows how hard you tried. He never wants you to think you should have done more. You are forever his mom. You are perfect. He won't leave your side. This is a new beginning where he can grow and you can too.

You can see why she is my earth angel. She gave me a glimmer of hope, even on my darkest day. You may ask how I knew any of that was true. Well I know Jillian and I know her gift to connect with angels and souls who have crossed over. I also know that she would never lie to me, especially about my son who had just died. If you need further convincing, she said that Zach told her all I ever wanted was for him to be happy and at peace. No one in the world knew that I always said that to Zach, except Zach.

I held onto that glimmer of hope that Zach wasn't "gone," even though I couldn't feel him yet. The next four days were a blur. I felt as though I was moving through a gray haze, as if the color had gone out of the world. Every morning when I woke up, there was that moment of blissful ignorance and then I would remember. I would remember that Zach had died and it was like a knife to the heart over and over again every morning. I wanted to stay in bed in the dark, but I could barely sleep anyway and during the days I wanted to hold it together in front of my boys, to be strong for them. As soon as my head hit the pillow at night, the tears would come for hours. Then I would finally pass out for a few hours and wake up at 5:00 am. It was an exhausting cycle.

There was never a doubt in my mind that I would do the eulogy at Zach's funeral. Who else could possibly speak about my Zach's life and the impact he had on this earth better than I could? I asked Peter if he wanted to do it with me and he said, "You're crazy." So every morning at 5:00 am when the house was quiet, I worked on my eulogy, editing and rewriting. It was one of those mornings when I got my first sign. I was looking out the picture window down onto the driveway, crying, when two deer walked up. Now we always have deer around because we live in the woods, but I had never seen deer walk right up to the cars and just stand there. It was a mama deer and her baby. They stood still and the mama deer locked eyes with me for a good ten minutes. Then they walked off together into the woods. Every cell in my body knew that this was a sign for me that Zach and I would always be together like the mama and baby deer. It was surreal.

People kept saying to me, "You're so strong." The truth is, when you lose someone so unexpectedly, you're still in shock for days. I suppose it is how we manage to function. Between the shock and the constant flow of people coming and going, somehow I kept going. There was no choice. The most important thing to me was my boys' well being. I worried about them so much. I knew how deeply this would affect their lives forever and I just wanted them to be able to move forward and have happy lives, despite the loss of their Zach. I wanted to be present for them. If I couldn't be okay, how could they?

There was so much to do. The day after Zach died, Peter and I had to meet with the funeral director and church director. Not only did we have to plan the wake, the funeral, the obituary, pick out a coffin and burial place, but we were still in Covid times so there was concern of a thousand people coming to the services. The funeral director suggested the local Tabernacle Church for the wake instead of the funeral home because it was large enough to hold more people and they could be spaced apart. Our church said we had to limit people at the funeral so we had to "invite" our close friends and family to the funeral. We were too overwhelmed with everything to sit down and create a list of who to invite to Zach's funeral, so unfortunately some of our close friends were not there.

We asked Father Joe Betti who was the former priest at Canisius High School to perform the funeral service. Zach and all the Canisius boys adored him. He met with us and we chose readings that Francine and Peter's cousin Michelle would be reading. We picked out music. Music is extremely important to Zach and me. More than anything, I wanted *Home* to be played.

As luck would have it, a boy named Ryan Downing reached out and asked if he could sing at Zach's funeral. Ryan was the cousin of our friends the Downings, he was a friend of Christopher, and he and Zach had a special relationship. In typical Zach style, there is a story behind it. Back in 2014, I got a call from Ryan's mom Angela. She wanted to tell me that Zach had saved Ryan's life and to thank me for having such a great kid. Petes was twelve at the time and had gone to the Bills stadium to watch Canisius play in the championship game. We sent Zach to pick him up but as soon as Peter got in the car, Zach saw Ryan getting beat up by a bunch of kids. Without hesitating, Zach jumped out of the car and single handedly started hitting guys and getting them off Ryan. There is literally a video of the whole thing. To this day, Angela says that Zach saved Ryan's life. How fitting for Ryan to sing *Home* for Zach.

My biggest job was picking out photos and music for the wake. The funeral home would make a video of the photos to music, but I also wanted all of the photos on boards. When my boys were little I had always put all of the photos into albums. After that, all of the photos have always been on my phone. My Covid project was developing all of those photos and putting them into albums. It was ironic. There I was a few months later, going through every album and ripping them all back out. My sister and brother were angels, helping me to glue all of them onto boards. It took days. There were seven giant poster boards of photos of Zach. His whole life fit onto seven poster boards. When I was going through all of those photos of him and he looked so happy, I wondered when he had begun to be in such pain. It was probably long before he had told us.

Being so busy helped get me through the week, but what helped even more was the kindness from our family and friends. The outpouring of love and support from our community was overwhelming. My friends all came over with food; some were delicious homemade dinners and some were dinners from our favorite restaurants. Hutch's was Zach's and my favorite restaurant. When Zach was young, I always brought him my jambalaya pasta leftovers. It became his favorite dish and soon enough, Hutch's became his favorite place for special occasion dinners. I even got the recipe for that pasta and would make it for him on his birthday. After he died, my friend Annmarie asked Hutch's to make a giant platter of it for us in honor of Zach. We ate it for days.

Our friends sent flowers and plants and gift cards. I received some of the most thoughtful and personalized gifts: a glass hologram ornament of Zach's face that hangs in my kitchen window, a wind chime with his name and birthday, a hurricane lantern with photos of him on every side, a "comfort" box filled with candles and a cozy blanket, bracelets, angels, the list goes on. Jillian had a star named for Zach and gave me a beautiful sun catcher that Zach wanted me to have. It hangs in my kitchen window and reflects beautiful colored lights all over the walls.

One of Zach's friends had spray painted "LIBZ" on a downtown building near the water right after he died. It was huge. Our friends, the Manns, took a photo of it and had it made into a glass print. It hangs in my kitchen. The Dowling family asked Canisius High School for Zach's #2 football jersey and they gave us both the blue and white jerseys, one for Peter and one for me. We laid it across Zach's coffin. I know he liked that. Perhaps my favorite gift was from Zach's Lily and Christopher's girlfriend McKenzie. They gave me a big stuffed "Pluto" dog with Zach's name and birthday on the dog tag.

My mailbox was stuffed to the brim with beautiful cards, every day for weeks. People took the time to write about Zach and why they loved him. What was really amazing was the kindness of strangers. People I didn't know reached out through Instagram and Facebook. I began to receive so many messages from people who shared a story about how Zach helped someone, or how Zach was kind to someone. One boy told me that he went to Canisius with Zach and he wasn't a friend of his, but Zach always smiled at him and said hello. He said that when he read Zach's posts about his struggles with mental health, it helped him feel less isolated in his own struggles. I literally received hundreds of messages like that.

Then something truly incredible happened. Zach had met so many people at treatment centers over the course of eight years. Many of them began to reach out to me to tell me that Zach had helped them, counseled them. Some even said that he had saved their life. We had no idea. All of the time that he had been in school to become a counselor and all that time he had spent alone in his room on the phone, he was counseling people.

I can't begin to explain how bittersweet it was for me to find out that while Zach was in some of his darkest times, he had helped others out of their darkest times. It was so overwhelming. Through my pain, I had deep gratitude for all that Zach had done to help others but I also couldn't help but feel how unfair life was. If he could help all of those people, why couldn't he help himself?? Yet I was beyond proud of him. I had always known that he was an exceptional human and a beautiful soul. His kindness and compassion and inclusivity towards all beings are what he will be remembered for. His courage to share his struggles in order to help others continues to help people today. Perhaps his brothers and friends will remember him most for his humor. Even when he was in so much pain, he strived to make others laugh.

Unfortunately six weeks after Zach died, my email was hacked and my Facebook and Instagram accounts were taken and I was unable to retrieve them. The worst part of it was that I cannot access the hundreds of messages that people had sent me and some of them I never even had the chance to respond to. I am so grateful for each and every message and story about my Zach.

The final thing we had to do was buy clothes for us to wear to the services. My friend Melissa picked me up and drove me to the mall to help me find a black dress for my son's funeral. Peter and I took the boys to a men's store to buy them suits and shirts and shoes. The sales people were so kind to us. At one point, I collapsed in a chair in disbelief when I was searching for the fourth suit and realized there were only three of them now. All of the pants needed to be hemmed so I had to bring the boys to the local tailor and ask her to hem six pairs of pants and my dress in a day. She was so kind to us and she said, "Yes, of course." The kindness of people literally kept me going.

CHAPTER TWENTY TWO

The day of Zach's wake arrived. Peter's fiancé Melissa asked if she could come over to give me a gift. She had a jeweler make matching necklaces for each of us, a gold chain with a tiny diamond "Z". I was overwhelmed by her thoughtfulness. I love it and I wear it every day. There was a viewing the night before and we were saddened to see that Zach didn't look like himself. We had donated his organ tissue so maybe that was why. My mom said, "I'm not even crying. That doesn't even look like Zach." Perhaps that happened to make it easier for all of us to see him like that. For me, Zach was already gone. He wasn't in that body.

The wake was the longest day of my life. We all lined up: Peter and me, our boys, Melissa, Keith, Peter's sister Carol, and my brother and sister. We stood for more than six hours while a steady stream of more than 1,500 people came to pay their respects. I felt so many emotions at once. We all had to wear masks so most people had to tell me who they were. The pain in their eyes hurt my heart. People hugged me and cried in my hair all night long. I felt like I was comforting many of them.

Unfortunately there is one thing that you learn quickly when going through deep grief is that some people will let you down. There were people who I thought I was close to that didn't come to the wake, perhaps because of Covid or because it was too hard for them. If you are in that situation, my advice is to forgive people. Immediately. Instantly. Grief takes up too much of our energy; there is no energy left for hurt and resentment. Also, forgiveness is really about healing ourselves.

More than anything else, I was beyond grateful for the outpouring of love from our family and friends and the entire community of WNY. I was particularly grateful to all of the young people who showed up for my sons. They came from all over: Florida, Ohio, Pennsylvania, and the list goes on. Zach's Lily, Christopher's McKenzie and Eric's Lily had been at our house every day to be a support for them. My boys are so loved and it made me happy to see their friends, classmates, teachers and coaches supporting them.

Nothing was harder for me that day than seeing Zach's friends. It was horrible to see the harsh reality of it on their faces. At one point, what appeared to be Zach's entire Canisius football team and coaches showed up. It had been seven years since they all played together, but they showed what a brotherhood truly is. It brought tears to my eyes when I saw them lined up and I was filled with gratitude.

At one point, a young girl came up to me who I didn't recognize. She was on the verge of tears and I asked her name. She had met Zach in treatment and she said that Zach had saved her life. TWICE. I was speechless. She said she had driven by herself from New Jersey to be there to say good bye to him. We hugged and cried. It became easy to recognize those that Zach had helped. They would walk forward hesitantly and I always had to ask their name and they would tell me their story of how Zach had helped them. There was a teenage girl who was escorted forward by her parents. She was shaking. She said that Zach had saved her life. She had met him at Brylin. Her parents couldn't even speak. They were on the verge of tears and I saw the look of fear in their eyes that this could have happened to them. And still could. I was so filled with gratitude that Zach had helped her, that he had helped so many. It was truly overwhelming.

One thing was for sure, Zach was so beloved. The day went on forever and we never had a chance to sit down or eat. We were completely exhausted, emotionally and physically. Then it was over and we had to say goodbye to Zach. It was the last time we would see his face. It was too awful to even put into words. I told him I loved him and thanked him for being such a wonderful son. I kissed him for the last time.

October 8th, 2020 was the day of Zach's funeral, the second worst day of my life. It was a beautiful fall day; the sun was shining brightly and the sky was azure blue. As we arrived at the church, our friend Tracey handed us homemade masks that she had made for us. They were plain navy and black masks with a gold "2" on them, Zach's football number at Canisius. It was another act of kindness that meant so much to us.

It was the most beautiful service I have ever seen, the way I had hoped it would be. I wanted it to be a celebration of Zach's life, and it was. Ryan began the service singing *Home* with his guitar and he sounded like an angel. I knew Zach loved it; it was the first time I felt his presence strongly. Of course he was there with us. Father Betti did a beautiful, personal service, including a sermon with an analogy to football which he had shared with the Canisius football team in the past.

When it came time for the eulogy, I felt myself shaking and I was nervous that I would not be able to get through it without breaking down and crying. Christopher had told us that he wanted to speak about Zach as well and we were astounded at his bravery. As Father Betti called us up, I suddenly felt a wave of complete calmness wash over me. I knew that it was Zach and that he was with me.

Christopher went first:

> *I don't really know how this is going to go, so bear with me. I told myself I wasn't going to get emotional either because I know Zach would have just called me soft. Where to start... I won't tell you about the fact that Z stole all my clothes, stole all my money, and embarrassed me in public the majority of time... because that wouldn't be appropriate. But on a serious note, my brother Zach. He truly was*

one of a kind. A one in a billion person. You will never meet a person with the same character and spirit that he had. He was the most spontaneous, selfless, and caring person I have ever met. But everyone here today already knows that about him. He could talk to anyone. Even people he didn't know.. he would greet them with a bright smile, a slap up, and a soft 'yeppp.' Zach cared about literally every person in his life, more than they could ever imagine. He wasn't just a big brother to Eric and Peter and me, he was a big brother to every one of our friends as well. He saw how much we cared about our friends and he made it a point to care about them and treat them like family as well. As I thought back on memories we shared together for a story to tell, I instantly thought of one that showed his true selflessness and care for others. A few years back, my dad had been out of town on vacation ... so obviously we had to throw a party together.. sorry Pops. The following day, we found out my mom was coming to the house to check if anyone was there and we knew we were done for. As we scrambled around trying to clean up and get everyone out, Z looks at me and says, 'I'm taking the heat.' I said bro, mom and dad both know that my friends were here and you can't. He responded with another, 'I'm taking the heat.' This continued for a couple minutes until he looked me directly in my eyes and said, 'Miami... Heat. I'm taking it.' (We all laugh.) At that point I had to just sit back and accept the fact that he was taking the blame for all of us. Although this story might not be the most crazy or interesting, it's special to me because it was the first time I truly understood how much he cared for me and how badly he wanted to protect my friends and me. This love and care he shared was directed mainly towards his two favorite little brothers, Eric and Peter, and if you're going to ask, yes... I was the least favorite. All he wanted was to see them excel in their respective sports and more importantly, for them to be happy in life. All he did was love and care for all those around him while never asking for it to be returned. As I continued to write this out, I realized how much of Zach I was really going to miss… his crazy obsession with 'The Office,' recording himself throwing footballs into basketball hoops, and even his snapchats singing along to his favorite Johnny Cash songs behind the wheel. If he were here right now, I would simply tell him thank you. Thank you for teaching me how to get the most out of life. Thank you for teaching me that making someone else smile can even make yourself feel good. Thank you for being my inspiration to keep on living every single day. And thank you for being the best big brother us three could have ever asked for. We love you brother, forever and always. Fly high Z.

He was funny, charming, and heartfelt. I was never as proud of Christopher as I was at that moment. It took so much courage to get up there and speak on this day when we were all in such raw pain, but he did it for Zach. I told him that he didn't have to stay up there with me because my eulogy was so long and emotional, so he went to sit down and I stood there alone. I felt myself waver without anyone there for support, but once again I felt my Zach with me.

The church was filled with people but because we had to limit how many people could come because of Covid, we were able to post a link to the funeral service for those who could not attend. What a godsend that was. Our friends and Zach's friends were able to watch the service from all over the country. It has almost 3000 views. Jillian was watching at home and she said that the light behind me was so intense, she had to turn her head away. It was Zach of course.

I won't write out my entire eulogy because it was quite long. I spoke of how grateful we were for the love and support from our community. I spoke about Zach as a boy who everyone loved. I talked about his love and adoration for his three brothers, his love of football, and his love of *Harry Potter*. I quoted Dumbledore and Sirius Black. I know he liked that.

Zach's friend Sam posted a beautiful tribute on his Instagram and I had asked him to read it. He said that he would rather I read it so I included it in my eulogy:

> *I really love this kid. He was special. He is special. One in a billion. He paid attention to every single person in the room. He made sure everyone was involved. An empath and an altruist. An old soul. He saw people for who they were, not for who he wanted them to be, and that's why he loved them. He knew how to get you to open up. He knew how to talk you off the ledge. No matter what he was going through, he always had a smile on his face, and so did you. Gave out an infinite amount of favors to everyone, and never asked for anything in return. He was loved by everyone who knew him and he never had a bad word to say about anyone. He had the right perspective. He knew that personal relationships were worth more than any currency or possession imaginable. While I know he finds solace in realizing how many people he touched, he would be heartbroken to see how many people are mourning his loss. He deserves to be celebrated.*
>
> *He struggled a lot these last few years, but he was determined to get back on track with school so that he could become a counselor, and become a positive influence in the lives of kids that struggled with mental health issues themselves. His first priority was always helping people, and we can't allow that to stop. I know nothing would make him happier than creating some sort of foundation for mental health to continue his mission when the dust settles, because he truly deserves to see that carried out. There's not a single*

person that I believe deserves happiness more than Z does.

There's so much more I could say, but if you knew him, you already know. If there's one thing I find comfort in, it's knowing he and Nolan are back together talking their shit with Bay right by his side, Johnny Cash bumping in the back. It was and will forever continue to be an honor to call you my brother Z.

I couldn't have said it better myself. He truly knew Zach. I ended my eulogy with:

As for me, I practice gratitude every day and here is what I am grateful for today: I'm so grateful Zach picked me to be his mom. Grateful for every day that we had with that beautiful soul. I'm grateful for all of the lives that he touched. I'm grateful for all of our family and friends. Grateful for Melissa and Keith for loving our boy, in the most difficult of circumstances. So grateful for Peter, because we've always been a team and neither one of us could have gone through all of this alone. Mostly, I'm grateful for my sons Christopher, Eric, and Peter who always lifted Zach up, and held him up there for so long.

I'd like to close with another Harry Potter quote: 'But know this; the ones who love us never really leave us.' Zach will always be with us. His light will shine through us. Fly high Zach-a-doo. I know you're with Little Grandma, Nolan and Bailey now. We know you're finally at peace but we will miss your beautiful smile SO MUCH.

I truly was so grateful in that moment for the people who came to the church that day to celebrate Zach's life and for my incredible family and friends. I was grateful for every message and text that I received, because even though I was in unbearable pain, I truly felt that love.

There is nothing more heart-wrenching than watching a funeral procession of parents following their child in a casket. It took all of my effort to get my legs to walk. Christopher had his arm around me and helped propel me forward. I would have liked to have seen every person in the church and thanked them for coming, but we piled into the car out of exhaustion. Normally we would have gotten to see everyone at the funeral brunch but we were not able to have a big gathering, so I regret not getting to talk to everyone.

Our long processional of cars made it's way to the cemetery. Peter wanted Zach to be in a mausoleum so we chose a pretty little cemetery ten minutes away. We had to do the service outside and while we waited for everyone to park and assemble, I couldn't believe how many people were there. I have never seen so many people assembled at a cemetery service before, and once again, I was grateful. It was such a testament to how loved Zach was. Just before the service started, in the silence, there was a flyover from a military plane. I smiled. A sign from Zach.

Not surprisingly, the funeral director had his own *Harry Potter* analogy. He spoke of the mirror that Harry could see his parents in. If you're not familiar with *Harry Potter*, both of his parents had died when he was a baby. Harry finds a magic mirror that he can actually see them in and then spends most of his time in the mirror. It's a heartbreaking scene. The funeral director reminded us, "Don't stay too long in the mirror." In other words, recall the memories fondly, but don't get stuck in the past; keep moving forward. I knew he was right and I vowed to do just that, but I have since learned that it is much harder than it seems. I am still working on that.

We watched the endless stream of people say their last goodbye to Zach and lay a flower on the casket. Then we said our final goodbye to Zach. My heart felt as though it were broken in half as I walked away from him. I walked away from his body, but I knew he wasn't gone. I had already felt his presence.

We had a very small and short brunch for immediate family and friends. And then it was all over.

CHAPTER TWENTY THREE

THE DAYS AND weeks after the funeral were the darkest days of my life. I thought that it couldn't get worse after the funeral but it did, for when the shock began to wear off and there were no more tasks to do, the harsh reality set in. The sheer disbelief of what had happened hit me hard. Everyone went back to living their life and I was left with the realization that THIS was my life now; that I would have to live out the rest of my life without Zach here on earth. I honestly didn't know if I could do that.

I entered into a place that was so dark, it scared me. I now knew how Zach had felt all of those years when he was suicidal. It was difficult to have hope; I thought that I would never feel joy or happiness again. How could I? I had had moments in my life of not wanting to be here on earth anymore (haven't we all?), but this was different. I just didn't know how I could possibly stay here. I didn't know if I could get through one more day, but of course I would have to because I could not cause Christopher, Eric, and Peter any more pain. They needed me and I used every bit of strength I had to get through each day. I didn't want them to worry about me at all. I had to show them by my actions that we were going to move forward somehow and live our lives to the fullest because we know that's what Zach would want. I didn't know how I was going to do that, but I would find a way because if I couldn't move forward, how could I expect them to move forward?

All of the tools that had helped me in the past were not helping now. I couldn't meditate at all because I would either cry or get really angry. I didn't have the energy for a yoga practice. I felt so heavy.

And then the guilt set in. I think that all bereaved parents, no matter how their child died, holds onto guilt. We are the parents. We are supposed to protect them and keep them safe. It is literally our job. Somehow we are supposed to protect them from death. Spiritually this is not true, but from the parents' perspective, this is how we feel. Especially losing our child to a drug overdose, even though we spent years trying to help him, we blamed ourselves at first. The thought "Why couldn't I save him?" circled around and around in my mind, especially in the middle of the night. I talked to Zach, "I'm so sorry I couldn't save you Zach!" and sobbed.

I texted Jillian and told her the truth of how badly I was doing and how I was feeling. While anger and depression are normal reactions to grief, I was suicidal as well. I had always had such strong spiritual faith, but now I felt lost. I didn't understand WHY?! Why didn't God answer all of our prayers? Why didn't He heal Zach? Why did this happen to us? Why did this happen to me? Zach would have helped so many people, so WHY was he taken?? I remembered how I always used to meditate and picture Zach holding his newborn baby and now that was never going to happen. I would never get to dance with him at his wedding. All of those dreams were shattered now.

I dug down deep and tried to take a step back and view it all from the spiritual perspective. Deep in my heart, I knew from all of the spiritual lessons that I had learned that it wasn't up to me to save him. He had to save himself. I also believed that it was "God's Will" or it wouldn't have happened, and I knew without a shadow of a doubt that Zach was happy and free now. He was "Home" and that did bring me comfort, but the human mom in me suffered still. I had much work to do in order to heal.

I texted Jillian: *Was this God's plan? Was this all decided before we came into this life?*

She responded:

- *Your souls chose this before you came.*
- *You knew that the transition that is occurring on earth would be occurring and many people would struggle. Because of this, you decided to come together as a team. Temporarily together to connect on earth. Then continue your work in tandem with him on the other side.*
- *You both also knew that you would get distracted from your purpose and that Zach leaving this earth would prompt you to start a quest to connect, that would in turn teach others how to also.*
- *You did not decide this recently. It was a decision before you came to earth.*
- *He will tell you the next step. Your job is to heal and find peace so you can hear and feel his guidance. Zach is going to continue to help so many through you.*

I asked if he was close by because I couldn't feel him.
She responded:

Sweetie, I don't think he's close by. I KNOW he's close by. Please never worry. He is 100% connected to your soul energy. The two of you are going to do amazing things. It is like you have your own personal angel soul, higher self to speak and collaborate with at all times. You will see... just wait. The connection between the two of you will be stronger than ever.

Then she told me that I would not be able to imagine the amazing thing that Zach and I would do together exactly a year from now. I couldn't imagine, but she gave me a glimmer of hope and I couldn't wait to see what it was! I wasn't feeling him around me because I was in such a dark place. I asked Zach to give me cardinals as a sign and all of a sudden, cardinals would pop up outside my kitchen window all the time, so I knew that Jillian was right and that Zach was always nearby. I wanted to feel that strong connection and hear him, so I vowed to do whatever it took for me to heal and move forward. It became my quest.

The six weeks after Zach died were the hardest six weeks of my life, but I made it through. I did very basic yoga poses and restorative yoga every day. I did breathing techniques every day, especially when I found myself spiraling down into that dark place. The "4-7-8 breathing technique" was my go to. It helped. Jillian had suggested that I get back to teaching my yoga classes and private sessions a couple weeks after Zach died because it was healing for everyone, and so I did. It took all of my energy, but it did truly help me. I researched movement with sound for grief. I tried anything that could possibly help me to heal.

Almost every day my wonderful friends took turns picking me up and taking me for a walk. It was a gorgeous October in Buffalo. Every day was sunny with a perfect blue sky and the vibrant colors of the foliage were so beautiful that it hurt my heart. How could the world look so vibrant and colorful when my heart felt so dark? Still, these walks were healing for me to be out in nature and talking with friends. My friends brought me back to life.

Nolan's mom Kim Burch was a huge help for me. Just to be in her presence was a comfort for me because she was the only one who understood what I was really going through. She was also an inspiration to me because she was living her life with joy. It had been six years since Nolan had died, but I at least had hope that I too could be happy again someday.

After you lose a child, you begin to hear an expression from other bereaved parents, "You've joined a club that you never wanted to join." Sadly, you do feel part of this horrible club, but it's also a support system. Every parent I knew who had lost a child reached out to me and of course I do the same thing now. Whenever I hear of a mom who has lost a child, I always reach out with a text or message telling her that the days after the funeral were my darkest days and that it WILL get easier. We turn around and give a helping hand to those who are just beginning this devastating journey. It is an unspoken vow.

Another thing that helped me get through the first couple months was that I read every single book I could find about Heaven and "signs" from the other side. This is what I wanted, the thing that kept me going. I knew that Zach wasn't gone. I knew that even though he wasn't here on the earth plane anymore, I could still connect with him because so many other people can and do!

Then one of my intuitive friends told me that Zach was telling her to give me a book that she had read called *Healing Grief* by James Van Pragh. (It's an excellent book!) Zach wanted her to show me a particular passage in the book that described a young man who had died and he was helping children cross over to the other side when they died. Zach wanted me to know that that's what he was doing, helping children and young people make the transition to the other side. I knew that it was true. Of course Zach's beautiful smile welcomed kids to the other side. I also knew that my friend wouldn't lie to me. This brought me so much comfort; I was overwhelmed with tears.

Right after Zach died, his cousin Jonathan asked Peter and me if he could put together a remembrance fundraiser dinner at Wanakah Country Club where they all used to do swim team together. Even while we were still in the hospital with Zach, Peter and I talked about starting a foundation in his name. It was a given. There was no question that we wanted to keep Zach's name alive and to continue his legacy of helping people. While I was so grateful to Jonathan for wanting to do this, it was so soon and I didn't know if I had the energy to face that many people only three weeks after Zach died. Still, we couldn't possibly tell him no since he was so adamant that he wanted to do this for Zach.

We had absolutely nothing to do with it. Our family just showed up. Jonathan had put together a lovely dinner, 100 of their former swim teammates, friends, and family had come and it raised $9000 towards our foundation which we hadn't even founded yet. It was overwhelming, but it was a clear sign that we were meant to do great things in Zach's name. Peter and I didn't have the energy to get the foundation started yet, but once again I had a glimmer of hope.

Six weeks after Zach died, Keith and I took a trip to Aruba for a week. His parents and brother and sister-in-law had traveled from Saratoga for Zach's funeral, which meant so much to me, and his parents had generously gifted us their Aruba time share. I didn't want to go… going on a vacation did not sound appealing and most days I barely had the energy to climb the stairs, much less pack for a trip and deal with Covid testing and requirements. However, I knew that it would be healing for me because the ocean is my happy place, and Keith really wanted to go, so off we went. It turned out to be a godsend.

I had been to Aruba before and it is my favorite island, but the first couple of days were very difficult for me. Without the distraction of my boys and teaching at home, I had only my thoughts to focus on. Being on a vacation brought up so many memories of vacations with my boys, and every time I saw a boy who resembled Zach, my heart hurt. Grief leaves us in such a vulnerable state. At any moment, something can trigger a memory and it feels like a sharp stab of pain to the heart. It can be debilitating.

To make matters worse, Keith and I had to have a brief meeting while we were there and when the woman asked how many kids I have, I froze. It was the first time I was faced with that question and I hadn't prepared my answer yet. Keith quietly answered "three" to save me from having to talk about Zach. I know he was trying to help, but I felt like I couldn't breathe. It felt as though we were dismissing his whole life, his whole existence. As painful as it was, it was a helpful situation for me to be placed in so that from that moment forward, I had my answer prepared. When people ask me how many kids I have or how old my sons are, I respond, "My son Peter is 21, my son Eric is 23, my son Christoper is 25, and my oldest son Zach is on the other side now. He died in October 2020." It's not easy for the person to hear of course, but I will not omit the truth of my Zach's existence in order to spare their discomfort.

A few days in, I was swimming in the ocean and Keith had gone up to the room. The beach was practically deserted because of Covid travel restrictions. Whenever I'm in the ocean, I face the horizon and swim and jump waves and completely lose track of time. At that moment, the thought came to me that I could just keep on swimming towards the horizon. I could swim until I was too tired to swim anymore and then I could give up and go see my Zach. I looked around; nobody was looking at me. No one would even notice me swimming out to sea. I started swimming as fast as I could toward the horizon. I was done with this life. I just wanted to see Zach. Then I remembered my boys. I could not, and would not, leave them without their mom. And so I turned around and swam back in. I knew I had the strength to stay in this life, but I just didn't want to.

I am not ashamed to admit any of that, but I am not proud of it either. It just was. It was a turning point for me. I knew I had to pull myself out of this darkness and that no one could do it for me.

From that moment on, the Aruba trip took a turn for the better. Everything changed. The next day when I was in the ocean, I allowed myself to feel the joy that I always feel in warm ocean water with the sun on my face. My heart felt lighter and I felt happier and as soon as that happened, I felt Zach. I felt his presence. I felt his energy with me as I jumped waves, the familiar energy of him when he was alive and he was sitting right next to me. I closed my eyes and I could see his beautiful face, so bright, as if he was lit up. "I love you Zachy." "I love you mom." I could hear him.

That was when I learned firsthand what I had been told by Jillian and what I had read about; we can connect better with our loved ones on the other side when we raise our vibration. VIBRATION. All energy resonates at a vibration, and all beings are energy. Our loved ones on the other side are of the highest vibration, the vibration of love. Our vibration is affected by many things: earth, the food and drink we consume, and our thoughts and emotions. Love, gratitude, joy, and compassion are high vibration. Fear, sadness, guilt, anger, regret, worry are low vibrational. So while it is normal to feel sadness and grief over the loss of a loved one, it also makes it harder for us to connect with them.

At that moment in the water when I was joyful, I felt Zach so strongly and then after that, the signs from him began to come. I was sitting on our balcony one day, reading a book about a dad trying to connect with his son on the other side. Suddenly a giant bird with human-like eyes came onto the railing and stared at me. We sat like that for at least 15 minutes while tears streamed down my face. I knew it was a sign from Zach. I KNEW with every part of my being that he was telling me he was with me and that he would give me signs, just like the dad and son in the book.

The next day, Keith and I went for a long walk on the beach, passing hotels and restaurants. As we passed a casual beach restaurant, a song was blaring from inside … Johnny Cash singing *Ring Of Fire*. We looked at each other and laughed. There are three songs that we all know are undoubtedly signs from Zach: *Home*, Phillip Phillips, *Ring Of Fire* or any Johnny Cash song, and *See You Again*, Wiz Khalifa with Charlie Puth. When I was picking out songs for the photo slideshow for the wake, the funeral director gave us a list that we had to choose from. When I showed the list to the boys, they each immediately pointed to *See You Again* from the *Fast and Furious* movies that they all used to watch together. That is their song for Z.

Ring Of Fire was from the movie *Walk The Line* which was one of Zach's favorite movies. Not only was he giving me a sign, it was a funny sign, having Johnny Cash playing when you'd normally hear island music. Typical Zach making me laugh. I would continue to see how funny he can be with his signs. The next day, people were playing music on the beach and *See You Again* came on.

Suddenly I noticed how a random "Z" would appear out of nowhere. I would look at my phone and a "Z" or "ZZZZZZZ" would look as if I typed it to someone, but I didn't. Zach was primarily known as "Z" to his dad, his friends, his brothers, and his brothers' friends. Over the course of his life, he had many nicknames: Zach-a-doo, then in football he was called Libs, and then when his brothers were all playing football, they were all called Libs so they became Z-Libs, C-Libs, E-Libs, and P-Libs. Christopher called each of them by their first initial. I know that Zach gets a kick out of giving us random "Z"s. I saw "Z"s everywhere on that trip.

Even though I was in deep grief and cried every day in Aruba, I also saw signs every day and every time I was swimming in the ocean, I felt Zach there with me. The most important thing about signs is that you have to believe them and the more you see them and believe them, the more signs you will get. As we returned home to Buffalo, I was hopeful that I would be able to continue to connect with Zach as I had on the trip.

CHAPTER TWENTY FOUR

In MY EXPERIENCE, grief does not come in stages. There are emotions that most of us go through after loss: shock, sadness, denial, depression, anger, the feeling of being overwhelmed, the list goes on. One day I would be in deep depression and then the next day, I would be really angry. Then I could have a day when I actually didn't cry that much, but back into depression the next day. There were no stages to get through; it was a constant roller coaster of emotions. One thing I know for sure is that everyone must grieve in their own way and what works for some, may not work for others.

When we returned home, the reality of it all hit me hard again and I felt myself slipping back into the darkness. Being away from my house and away from people knowing about Zach everywhere I went, was freeing and I felt like I could breathe in Aruba. Back at home there were reminders everywhere. I have photos of Zach in every single room in my house. I have a "shrine" of sorts in the family room with his photo from the wake, his handprint, memory candle, and other gifts. Zach's bedroom is at the top of the stairs and I have to walk by it several times a day. It is exactly as he left it. I know that someday it will be time for me to clean out his room, but I am not ready yet. Back then, I would sit on his bed to feel close to him and just cry by myself. He had left three dirty shirts in his hamper and I have kept them that way because they still smell like him. It was all I had left of him. That, and a "NYC" hoodie that he begged me to buy him when we went to New York. I wear it every morning when I wake up to feel close to him.

The cold, gray winter was beginning and the holidays and Zach's birthday were upon us. I struggled every day to fight the waves of excruciating pain that came unexpectedly, at any given moment. A song that came on in the car could be a sign from Zach that would make me laugh, or it could spur a memory that would make my heart hurt and instantly bring tears to my eyes. Most days I felt exhausted and heavy. I felt broken.

Although Christopher had moved to Tampa, he had only been there a week when Zach died so he hadn't started a new job yet. Thankfully, he was able to stay with us for a few months before he went back. He needed to be with his family. He too appeared to be depressed and I worried about him. Eric was right back at work and Peter was back in school so at least they were busy. Having them all in my house saved me. I went through the daily motions of teaching, cleaning, cooking, but their presence in the house lifted me up, just as they had lifted Zach up. Peter's senior football season had been postponed until spring because of NYS Covid restrictions, so the high schools did some flag football games in the interim which gave us something to do. It would have been wonderful for Peter and our family to have had a real football season to give us a distraction.

I know that my boys struggled with guilt about Zach and of course they had absolutely NO reason to feel guilty about anything, but feeling guilty is normal when overdose is concerned. Christopher felt guilty that he wasn't here. Eric and I could have brought Zach to my house that night and if we had, he probably wouldn't have overdosed. Peter was mad at his dad because he had switched nights and the boys would have been with Zach at his house. The fact is, there were a hundred things that could have gone differently, but we will never know if it would have changed anything. I told them that even if we had prevented him from overdosing that night, we couldn't have prevented it every day. What is meant to happen will find a way.

I suggested counseling to all of them. They all had had the same school counselor at Orchard Park High School and she had become a friend to our family. She got special permission for Eric to be able to come in, even though he had graduated. I believe that she helped Eric and Peter greatly. She reiterated how helpful exercise can be for grief and overall mental health, and Eric began going to the gym again everyday which I know has been extremely beneficial.

I had a pit in my stomach as Thanksgiving approached, our first holiday without Zach here. My only goal for Thanksgiving and Christmas was to have my family for dinner as I always have, to keep our family traditions alive. I had attended a support group for bereaved parents a few weeks before and some of the parents, even years after their child had died, were not able to move forward. Some didn't even celebrate holidays anymore. I could see how easy it would be to fall into that category. Hosting the holidays sounded exhausting to me, but I vowed that we would not alter our traditions because Zach wasn't here. It wouldn't be fair to my boys. I wanted to show them that our lives would continue without Zach. We would somehow move forward. I wanted them to know that they will always be as important to me as my son who isn't here. I refused to "go down with the ship" that was Zach. I could see how easy it would be for me to be lost forever in that grief and darkness, to be a ghost of my former self. No matter what it took, I would not let that happen.

Most importantly, I just wanted all of us to be together for the holidays. It was not an easy Thanksgiving. It was solemn to be sure, but I was thankful for my sons and for my family, and for my Zach who was always close by.

Then it was December. Christmas has always been my favorite time of year, but when I brought my first baby boy home four days before Christmas, it became purely magical. Since then, Christmas was always intertwined with memories of Zach. I decorated the house as I always do, but a day that normally brings me so much joy was so bittersweet. I was caught off guard when I came upon my foyer decoration and memories of the day Zach was born came flooding in. Our moms had sent a beautiful gold sleigh filled with greens and ornaments and bows to the hospital. I loved it so much that I had it redone with artificial greens so that I could keep it forever. I cried as I remembered the day that Zach was born. We decorated the tree and hung ornaments that Zach had made when he was young. I have an ornament of his first Christmas. It was impossible to believe that he wasn't here.

As Zach's birthday approached, I knew that we needed some kind of distraction in our lives. When Bailey died, I knew without a doubt that I would get another dog, but I needed time to mourn her. If there was ever a time for a new dog in the house, this was it. I really wanted an adult golden retriever who needed a home but after Covid, dogs everywhere had been adopted. I began to search for a golden retriever puppy. I put feelers out to all the dog people I know and searched online locally but there was a waitlist everywhere. I broadened the search and we finally found a puppy in Ohio. Eric and I planned to drive together to pick her up (I wanted a female) and I was literally about to put the deposit down, when one of my yoga students called me. She had a friend who worked at a vet in Rochester and said there might be a puppy available.

I didn't know what to do. We had this puppy already picked out, but an hour drive would be easier than a four drive to Ohio. The next morning I called the number I had been given. The woman explained that they are a family that breeds their own goldens and the mama "Gabby" had just had a litter. They were all adopted except for three males that they decided to keep. One of the puppies was blind so they wanted to keep a brother pup for companionship. She had mentioned at her vet that keeping three of the puppies may be too much since they now had six dogs, however she told me that they had changed their minds. She and her husband decided to keep all three puppies. She said that she was sorry to get my hopes up and then she said, "Tell me your story."

I told her that I had four sons and that Zach had died two months before. I told her that our Bailey had died six months before that and we desperately wanted a new dog. There was a moment of silence and then she said, "Of course the puppy is yours if you want him." I couldn't believe it, but we still had a hold on the puppy in Ohio, so in my head I asked my angels and Zach, "Please give me a sign." Then she said that she also has four sons (sign #1). She said that one of her dogs is named Bailey (sign #2). And just in case I needed further proof that this was our dog, she said that her name was Mary (Peter's mom's name and sign #3).

Mary said that I could pick him up immediately, even the next day. The next day was Zach's birthday and I told her that maybe that would be a lot since our family had a full day planned, including meeting early at the cemetery. Again she paused. "Don't you HAVE to bring him home on your son's birthday??" I laughed. Yes of course I had to bring him home on Zach's birthday. It was clearly meant to be.

So very early the next morning, Keith and I drove to Rochester to pick up my new puppy. When we pulled up to the house, Mary was outside waiting for us with "Carli." He was the biggest ten week old puppy I had ever seen. As I walked toward him and our eyes met, I started to cry. Yes this was my puppy. It was love at first sight. He even had a white marking on his forehead which reminded me of Harry Potter's scar. Zach had a similar scar on his forehead from when he had stitches when he was three. He cuddled on my lap all the way home.

As we pulled into the driveway my three boys were standing in the window waiting for their new puppy. I will forever be grateful for that moment when they met their new dog because it was the first time I had seen them genuinely happy since before Zach had died. I said that we had to change his name and they said in unison,

"Blue! His name is Blue."

I asked, "Why Blue? Because Zach's favorite color was blue?"

They said, "Because Zach always used to say, 'You're my boy, Blue!' from the movie *Old School.*"

I laughed. Of course. And so his name is Blue. I call him Blue boy. He was a godsend that day, and every day since. I don't know how I would have gotten through the past years without him. There is no way Zach didn't orchestrate this. He knew it was the only way to bring his mom and his family joy on that incredibly difficult day. Peter and the boys and I brought balloons to Zach's grave. Then the whole family came over for pizza and watched the Bills game at my house. McKenzie and Zach's Lily and his best friend Danny came too. Blue reveled in the love from everyone.

The Bills won that day, capturing their first AFC East title since December 30th, 1995, eleven days after Zach was born. Zach's boy Josh Allen ran in two touchdowns. The day had Zach written all over it. He would have been 25 years old that day. I talked to him before I went to sleep. He is always the first soul I talk to every morning ("Good morning Zach") and the last soul I talk to at the end of every day ("Night Zach. Love you"). That night I said, "Happy birthday Zach! I hope you enjoyed your party." Of course I knew that he had been right there with us all day, especially when the Bills won. I thought I heard him say, "Thanks mom. I did."

Christmas was difficult without Zach, but we got through it. I always have the boys for Christmas Eve dinner with my family and they go to Peter's house for Christmas dinner. I went through the motions, but there were so many pangs of sadness. It had become our Christmas Eve tradition to watch *The Replacements* after dinner, so we did. There was a palpable void without Zach there that we could all feel.

On Christmas morning, I took the traditional photo of the boys in front of the Christmas tree. The three boys held Blue with a big red bow around his neck. It was the first time I could bring myself to take a picture of them without Zach. My heart ached. I wondered if it would ever get easier to see them together without Zach.

That cold, gray winter reflected how I felt inside. Christopher moved back to Tampa. I celebrated my first birthday without Zach here. He gave me a cardinal outside my window that morning, of course. I wanted to connect with Zach easier and feel his energy more. I knew I had to raise my vibration to do that, but didn't know how to pull myself out of the darkness. It was difficult going anywhere and seeing the looks of pity on people's faces. I had talked to a mom whose son had been gone for ten years and she said that she still couldn't be around people's "normal" conversations. I now knew what she meant; to be around other moms who were having normal conversations about their lives and their kids was painful. It obviously wasn't anybody's fault. It just was.

I also had to take a break from social media. While I was certainly happy to see friends' kids traveling, graduating, getting engaged, getting married, it also brought on waves of sadness and complete disbelief that my Zach would never be doing those things. I truly wondered if I could ever be happy again. It didn't seem likely.

However, a few months after Zach died, there were small shifts, small glimmers of light. Sue, Kerry, and I were out for dinner for my birthday and Sue brought up the most ridiculously funny memory from high school and I laughed so hard, I almost fell off my chair. It felt so good to laugh that hard again.

Around that time, I came across the movie *Little Women* on tv one night. *Little Women* was my favorite book as a child and I have seen every movie rendition. This time when I watched, it startled me that my life had so many parallels to *Little Women*. They had four girls and I had four boys. All four of the girls had an extremely closely bonded relationship, just as my boys did. They lost their beloved Beth and we lost our beloved Zach. What struck me the most was the last scene when they are celebrating their mom's birthday, years after Beth had died. The mom's three daughters are now all married and her grandchildren are all running around, and everyone is happy. At that moment, I realized that we would have happy times ahead. There would be weddings, and babies, and someday I would feel joy again. It gave me hope.

I spoke with Jillian about the fact that I was still in so much pain and darkness. She had a good analogy. She had been extremely ill and she said that when she slowly started to heal, she would have one day a week that was a tiny bit better. Then after awhile, two days a week were a little bit better. Eventually, there were more good days than bad. She suggested that

that's what would happen for me. That made sense to me and that also gave me hope. From that point forward, I tried to really notice when I had a day (or even an hour) when I wasn't in pain, so that I could take note of when those days were coming more frequently.

The first rule of healing that I learned for myself was to listen to my heart and only do what felt good to me. One of the things that didn't feel good was drinking alcohol of any kind. I am not a big drinker, I would say I'm a lightweight actually, but I would have wine on the weekends. After Zach died, I was not drawn to alcohol at all. While it sounded appealing to numb the pain, I knew that I would have to feel the pain full force in order to heal it. Additionally, alcohol is a depressant so the few times I drank in those first few months, I felt suicidal.

I also couldn't watch any tv shows or movies that were dark in any way. I was dark enough inside; I didn't need to add to it. Also in regards to vibration, alcohol lowers your vibration and so does watching dark shows. I was trying to raise my vibration. I watched my favorite romantic comedies: *It's Complicated, Something's Gotta Give, Sweet Home Alabama, 13 Going on 30*, and *The Holiday* over and over. I watched episode after episode of *Schitt's Creek*. I started watching *Gilmore Girls* on Netflix and it became my obsession. I wanted to live in *Stars Hollow* where nothing bad ever happens; nobody has cancer and nobody dies unless they're over 80. Sooki and Paris made me laugh in every scene. I watched all seven seasons, cried when it was over, and then started from the beginning again. My family made fun of me of course, but it felt like a warm hug when I watched that show.

I became very selective about where and when I socialized. If I had plans to go to a dinner or an event and then just couldn't deal with making small talk that day, or just didn't have the energy, I cancelled. Without any guilt. I became very good at discerning what felt good to me and what didn't, and it soon became clear to me how often I had not been following my inner guidance in my life before losing Zach. Jillian pointed out to me that this was self love. I was putting myself first. It was interesting that I had to lose my son in order to really allow myself to follow what makes me happy.

I continued to practice yoga every day. I continued doing breathing techniques whenever I felt myself spiraling downward. Jillian and I talked about allowing myself to grieve and honoring that human part of myself, but trying not to get "stuck" in the grief. Some days I felt very stuck. When I found myself feeling that way, the quickest way I found to raise my vibration was playing one of my favorite songs. Mantras also helped; also listing five things I was grateful for. Soon enough I was able to start meditating again which really helped to set the tone of my day. Another helpful hint from Jillian was to raise my vibration before I meditated (like playing a favorite song first), so I was starting from a higher vibration rather than starting at a lower vibration and "locking it in."

I read somewhere to try and find the light in the darkness. I worked very hard to try and find light. Over time, it did get easier.

CHAPTER TWENTY FIVE

In THE PAST three years since Zach died, I have had many readings with psychic mediums to connect with Zach. Every single reading was spot on and I knew that Zach was there giving me messages. I recorded all of them. My first reading after Zach died was with Krow Fischer, who channels "Red," who is a guide from the "Council of Elders" on the other side. (I know that sounds crazy but it is true.) I had readings with Red while Zach was alive and he gave me some helpful advice for him. Three months after Zach died, my sister Kerry and I had our first reading with Red, with Zach on the other side.

> Red: *It's a really loving universe. Zach was tucked into support as soon as he crossed over. He's a pretty quick study, isn't he?*

We laughed. Yes.

> Red: *It's not easy to be born; it's not easy to be on earth.*
>
> *He wants you to know the addiction came because of the mental illness.*
>
> *He says he hears people say that it was the addiction that killed him. He says no, it wasn't the addiction that killed him.*

Yes. I knew that.

> Red: *It was exhausting being in his mind.. nonstop.. like being on a treadmill that was going at high speed and he couldn't get off. Like there were squirrels running up and down inside of him. The drugs gave him moments of peace, like he could just catch his breath.*

> *Some people on earth who are going through a similar situation feel very alone, but he didn't. He knew he had so much love and support from his family. He knew that. He really knew that.*

> *He wants to be able to offer support to others. He was a really good counselor, wasn't he? Those are services he has offered in many lifetimes.*

(Not surprising.) I asked who he saw first when he crossed over.

> Red: *Mary, his grandma, was the first face he saw when he crossed over and she said to you, 'I've got him. Don't worry.'*

(Yes. I heard that.)

> Red: *He completed his transition over after that.*

(That's why I still felt him in the hospital room.)

> Red: *He felt support from both sides. You were talking to him when he was in the coma. He heard you. And when you knew it was time to let go of him, that was really brave on your end. We really want to acknowledge your bravery. You knew it was going to hurt you, but you chose to put your energy into what was best for him. Even though you knew it was going to break you. We want to acknowledge that. You showed soul maturity and you showed what unconditional love looks like.*

> *And he is so sorry to have put you through that moment. He is so sorry. He put you through a lot in this life. The person*

he loved the most, he hurt the most. But you know him.. always an optimist. He says, 'I will make this up to her.'

He wants you to know that he really tried.

(Yes. I know that.)

Red: *People believed that if he could only fix the addiction, he would be okay. If someone has a damaged hip, nobody will say anything if they take painkillers, but if it's a psychological problem, you're not supposed to take painkillers. Nobody was offering a solution. They told him that he can't use the things that help, but nobody offered another way to help. He tried meditation, but he just couldn't get his mind to slow down. He was going to rehab and doing the work for the sake of his family, but he didn't feel like it was helping him.*

Me: *How can I connect with him better?*

Red: *How did you connect with him before he was born? You knew him. You knew his energy... 'Oh it's you! I'm so happy you're coming!' Before he was incarnate and after he was incarnate, that relationship and connection is constant. That bond is there. It's a primal bond and that's how you connect. You know his responses back when you talk to him. Even though you're in a place of deep grief, that bond is there.*

You have a pretty clear connection with him. Ground yourself in your certainty please. It is difficult for them to communicate when they send forth the energy and then the person "bats it back." People think that they must be making it up, or are worried that others will think they're crazy. Recognize that this is a human gift; your ancestors used to communicate with their ancestors all the time. Then it became forbidden. Recognize that this is a natural human ability.

Have confidence that it's normal and natural to be talking to my son who I love. The more you practice, the easier it is.

Zach is referencing 'hugging.' (I will explain later.)

Red: *A lot of prayers came through for him. In the halfway place between earth and spirit, souls can feel that love and support; it feels like warmth and light and caring. It bathes them. He had so much love and support for him, he felt it. He was very loved and he knows he was loved.*

You on earth have the hard part. You are left to mourn.

He wants to get strong and he wants to be a support for you for the rest of your life.

I asked what else Zach would like to say.

Red: *He loves you. The whole life of support. Even times when it got really frustrating... he knows he was frustrating. He knows that. He tried his best. He just couldn't do it, even with all the love and support he had. It is often believed on earth that it is family environment and trauma and tragedy that cause all the problems, but that's not always the case. He had so much love and support from his whole family. He had a mother who never stopped believing in him. No matter how many times he let her down. She never stopped. That carried him through. He did not lose his belief in himself. He did not fall into self hatred. It would have been so easy for him to fall into those dark places.*

He wants to thank you for that. Even when you were frustrated, he would see you calm yourself down and then try again. He so appreciates that. He felt so much of the family's energy was directed at him and he didn't want that.
He's so sorry to let you down.

Me: He didn't let me down! He was a wonderful son.

Red: *He still is. And he's going to be zipping star to star through the universe in no time.*

He says, 'Thank you for the love and support.'

It is important that you realize that he was your son in this lifetime and you worried about him in this lifetime. Rightly so, you worried about him when he was alive. Rightly so. You don't have to do that anymore. You don't have to worry about him anymore. He has support and he has as much love as you gave him. It's over. And you did a really good job. He came through all of this without self hatred. If he was there, his hands would be on your hands and he would look into your eyes and he says, 'You can let go of all your worry about me now. Let go. Let go of the fear and the concern and the worry. Don't worry about me anymore. I'm fine. I've got everything I need and I've got your love.'

When you let go of that, you're left with the love and the joy and the missing him.

If you could see him now, you would see that big, shining, searchlight of a smile coming at you. And boy he could really blast those smiles, couldn't he.

Oh yes he could. I was overwhelmed with tears throughout the entire reading, but it was so helpful and healing for me. When you have a really good reading, it's so incredible that you know without a shadow of a doubt that your loved one is there. I knew that those messages were from Zach, that he was right there. I felt him. I could feel Zach's energy with us. Everything Red said was 100% true.

I now knew that I wasn't crazy for thinking that I could hear Zach talk to me. Now, when I talk to him and hear his response back in my head, I accept and believe it. I talk to him all day long. He must tire of me!

In the reading, Zach also acknowledged how I "hug" him. When I meditate, I picture white light coming into my heart center and then the white light spreads through my body and then expands to an egg shape surrounding me. Then I ask Zach to come into the white light and I picture him, I can feel him. I imagine myself hugging him with all my love and whenever I do that, I feel Zach's energy through every cell of my body. It feels as if he's sitting next to me, except it is right through me. It feels like pure love. Zach acknowledged that "hugging" and described it as if our energies are merging. Of course I do this every day and every time it is so powerful, I have tears streaming down my face.

Just to be clear, in case you are doubtful, Krow would obviously have no knowledge of any of this that takes place between Zach and me now, or what took place when he was alive and at the time of his death. There was never any doubt in my mind that Zach was at the reading. Red and the council also spoke about several things that happened in the hospital that were completely accurate.

Probably the most helpful information for me was to accept signs from Zach, without doubting them. If you see something and you feel that it could be a sign, then it is! I had certainly been seeing signs from Zach before then, but I sometimes allowed doubt to creep in and I now opened up to truly believing in all of the signs. You have to be open to see the signs or you won't see them.

Signs. I could probably write an entire book about the signs that Zach has given me. He is very good at it and true to his personality, they are often funny and make me laugh out loud. I've always asked him for cardinals, which in a subsequent reading he told me are "generic" but I ask, so he gets them to me. Ha! I had never noticed cardinals around my house before Zach died, but now they practically live here. They are outside my kitchen window, outside my bedroom window, and almost every time I am writing this book at my kitchen table, there is one in my backyard or on my deck. Many times a cardinal will whiz by my windshield as I'm driving. I have been on walks with Blue in my neighborhood and had cardinals follow me tree to tree. This morning I was walking Blue and not paying attention, and a cardinal flew right towards my face. So funny.

I also ask Zach to give me bluejays. They are my favorite bird, but I had never seen one in my neighborhood before. Until now. If I'm having a bad day or even if I just say, "Zach, can you please give me a bluejay today?" I will see one. Or sometimes I will see the bluejay on a bus or on a card. He has fun with it. One day Blue and I were walking and a cardinal and a bluejay flew tree to tree together as we walked. I read that bluejays and cardinals usually aren't seen together, but Zach made that happen. Recently I was having a sad day and I saw multiple bluejays fly into a tree. I thought it odd to see more than two, and then they flew to the next tree. One, two, three, four bluejays flying together. Four bluejays for my four boys. I always say, "Thanks Zach. Love you."

Writing this book has not always been easy. Writing about Zach's dark days made my heart heavy and sad and whenever I was writing about it, there would be a cardinal on my table outside my window. When I wrote about the day that Zach died, and was reliving it all, it felt like I was right back in it. I was huddled on my kitchen table, sobbing, and I felt Zach's energy surrounding me, like he was hugging me. It felt like pure love surrounding me. Something caught my eye and I saw a giant bluejay on the table outside, looking at me. Zach was telling me that he was with me.

I would say that he gives me the most signs through songs, which is no surprise since we both love music. As I mentioned earlier, he knows that the songs that remind us of him are *Home, See You Again*, and Johnny Cash songs. That March, I took Peter to visit the University of Tampa because he was looking to attend there in the fall. Christopher and I were waiting for Peter outside a restaurant, so we began walking alongside a marina with beautiful boats on one side and expensive condos on the other side. Christopher stopped and laughed. "Do you hear that?," he said. There was a tiny bbq restaurant in the middle of the condos and we could hear *Home* playing from inside. Zach making us laugh again.

In addition to all of these songs, Zach gives me my favorite songs, just to lift my mood. Everywhere. All the time. My favorite songs are: (don't judge)

- *In Your Eyes,* Peter Gabriel
- *The Prayer,* Celine Dion and Andrea Bocelli
- *Dancing Queen,* Abba
- *Viva La Vida,* Coldplay
- *September,* Earth, Wind and Fire
- *DJ Got Us Fallin In Love,* Usher
- *Where is the Love,* Black Eyed Peas
- *Raise 'Em Up,* Keith Urban featuring Eric Church
- *Nessus Dorma,* Andrea Bocelli (must be what Heaven sounds like)

Zach always knew that these were my favorite songs, perhaps because I have always yelled out, "My song!" whenever any of them came on. He knows that all of these songs put me in an instant good mood. As you can see, they are all old songs but somehow I hear them on the radio, in a store, on tv, or mysteriously playing on my phone without me selecting it.

I always have a current "favorite happy song." Currently it's *Calm Down,* Rema and Selena Gomez (one of Zach's favorites). Of course he always knows my current favorite happy songs and they mysteriously come on when I am feeling down. He also knows that any Journey song makes my heart happy and brings me back to senior year of high school when life was easier and I was oblivious to the sorrow that lie ahead.

He gives me songs that remind me of him. Eminem's *Lose Yourself* always reminds me of his football days; it would play as the team came out onto the field. Of course he gives me songs from *The Lion King.* He plays *I Will Survive* by Gloria Gaynor from T*he Replacements* movie and *Ain't No Mountain High Enough* by Marvin Gaye from *Remember the Titans;* two of his favorite movies that he would watch with his brothers.

Zach and I both love Harry Styles' music. I clearly remember the first time we heard *Night Changes.* We were driving and it came on the radio and we were both silent through the whole song and then looked at each other and nodded. "Good song!" He gives that song to me all the time and of course I know it's from him. I know that he is giving me a message through the song:

"Everything that you've ever dreamed of, disappearing when you wake up. But there's nothing to be afraid of, even when the night changes. It will never change me and you."

It's haunting. But I know that Zach is telling me that our bond will never change. He's not going anywhere. He's always close by.

Perhaps the funniest sign is that I see Zach's car all the time. Not his actual car, but one that looks just like it. He had two cars in his life, the first was an old silver Ford Explorer and then he had an old silver Chevy Trailblazer. They were the old boxy shape and they looked very similar, both beat up with lots of scratches and dents from all of Zach's OCD related fender benders. These are not cars that you see around much anymore, however I see them ALL the time. It makes me laugh out loud.

When Zach was a baby, I used to sing *You Are My Sunshine* to him. The reason I sang that song was that Peter's 10 year old cousin Erik died when Zach was two weeks old and we went to the funeral. It was the first time I went to a child's funeral and it was horrific, especially having a newborn baby at home. Erik had requested that we all sing *You Are My Sunshine* at his funeral so we all stood in the packed church and sang. It was a dark January day, but as we sang, the sun began to shine brightly through the big stained glass window. It was beautiful. I went home and immediately began singing that song to Zach. Whenever I sang it, I changed the last line to "Please don't take my Zachary away." My throat would catch every time I sang that. Did my soul know what was coming? I don't know, but my throat never caught when I was singing songs to my other boys. I now see *You Are My Sunshine* everywhere. It can be on a sign or on my Instagram feed. I can see it on a necklace or hear it on a commercial. Of course it is Zach.

And of course Zach gives me elephants. His beloved elephants. One day I was having a really sad day and when I was walking Blue, I passed a truck with a giant baby elephant on it. So funny. You may think that all of these things can be purely coincidental and random. All I can say is that when Zach gives me a sign, I KNOW it is a sign from him. If you don't open up to the signs all around you, you'll miss out on the magic of connection with your loved one on the other side. It brings me so much comfort knowing he is there.

Zach gives my sister Kerry lots of signs as well. He gives her "Z"s everywhere. They also have the music connection. She loves rock music and right after Zach died, she started hearing songs from ZZ Top and Led Zeppelin, the Z bands. The funny part is, Kerry never liked Led Zeppelin or ZZ Top, but Zach is in charge and he gives her the Z bands! She also asked Zach to give her songs from *The Replacements* and *Twilight*, movies that she would watch with us over the years. He gives her those songs all the time.

He gives his best friend Danny signs all the time. He also gets "Z"s from Zach, as well as the number 19, Zach's birthday. One day his mom and sister were visiting him in California and they all went to get LOVE tattoos together. When they came out, they did a group hug and as Danny turned, he saw a giant billboard that said, "Yepp."

Zach and his friends used to always say "Yepp" and of course all of Zach's brothers and their friends picked it up. Zach became known for his "Yepp." He even named his landscaping company Yepp Landscaping. They all just laughed. Zach must have approved of their tattoos.

Zach's dad and his wife Melissa were getting remembrance tattoos for Zach in Arizona and Peter said Bob Marley came on while he getting his. He said that he knew it was Zach.

Tattoos. Not one person in our family had a tattoo before Zach died. Zach always wanted to get the tattoo that his friends had for Nolan: "NMB," but his OCD wouldn't allow it. It would never be perfect enough or symmetrical and it would drive him crazy, so he never got one. I never had a desire for a tattoo. I thought they were cool but didn't really want one. Peter felt the same way.

After Zach died, that all changed. I knew I wanted something permanently on me that reminded me of Zach, that reminded others of him, and that honored his memory. We all did. Christopher and Eric went first and they went together. Christopher found something that Zach had written in his journal from Sierra Tucson, "Don't let anyone make you feel little."

He had that tattooed across his forearm in Zach's handwriting. It's eerie; it looks like Zach wrote on his arm. Zach had very distinct messy printing. Eric had the day Zach died tattooed on his forearm in roman numerals with a Z under it. They are both beautiful and I cried when I saw them. Peter and Melissa went next. Peter has *Fly high Z* on his wrist and Melissa has *Z;* on her wrist. Then my sister and I went. I have *Zach* tattooed on my forearm in his handwriting. It looks like he wrote his name on my arm and it makes me happy whenever I look at it. Kerry has a Z with a heart.

Immediately after Zach died, his cousins and friends began getting tattoos for Zach and sending me photos or posting pictures of them. It was interesting that at that point, there were no two alike. Every single person got something that was personal to them. Lily also found some notes in a journal in Zach's room and has *it'll be okay* tattooed on her arm in his handwriting. Nolan's sister Alex has *Yepp*; One of my boys' friends has *Until the next slap up... Yepp*. Another has a Z with an angel wing. There are variations of tattoos with #2 (his football number) and Zs and angel wings and Yepp. I absolutely love seeing all of the tattoos. I know Zach loves them. He has mentioned it in several readings.

One day, because Zach's Instagram was still open on my phone, I got a notification that he was tagged in a post by his friend Drew, who I never met. He lives in Missouri. It was a picture of a *Yep* tattoo on his ring finger and he wrote:

> *Vena Amoris/vein of love: The vein that runs directly from the vein on your left finger to your heart.*
>
> *'Yep,' a simple 3 letter word, that will never come out of my mouth unnoticed. During my time in mental health treatment, I made a dear friend named Zach. Zach and I had a lot in common, one of those things being the inability to open up when we aren't doing good. Zach had a catch phrase of saying yep, and even had a landscaping business named 'Yeppp Landscaping.' We both understood how overwhelming it can be to constantly have people checking in*

on you and asking how you're doing, but we still wanted to check in on each other every day. We eventually came up with the plan to talk once a night on the phone just about our days, and to text 'yep' each morning so we knew the other had made it through another night.

On October 2nd, 2020 I didn't get that text back. I found out what I already knew later in the day, that I had lost a good friend, and the world had lost a great man. I'd give anything for one more phone call or pizza on the beach, and I know I will get that one day. But for now, I choose to live, and live the way that he did. With his heart on his sleeve, and arms always open to help another even when he was drowning.

Hug your people tight while you can, tomorrow is AL-WAYS a blessing.

It was one of those stabs of pain that came out of nowhere. I cried for this young man, thinking about him not getting a "yep" text back from Zach and knowing what had happened. Zach had so many friends, so many people that loved him that I didn't even know. He had helped so many people that I didn't know about. Every few months, I would find out about another friend that he had helped. I had to ask, "Oh Zach, why couldn't you help yourself???"

Of course I reached out to Drew and he responded:

Your son helped me through some of the hardest nights, I can't thank you enough for the man you raised. He might not be of this world anymore but I've definitely felt him when I needed him.

That wouldn't be the last time I would hear that from one of his friends.

CHAPTER TWENTY SIX

As we approached the six month anniversary of Zach's death, Peter's senior year finally went into full swing and it was a welcome distraction for all of us. They squeezed the varsity basketball season in, but we still had NYS Covid restrictions. Spectators were not allowed except for two people per player. We had to sit on tape markings on the bleachers to keep everyone spaced apart and the players had to wear masks while they were playing. It was a let down of a senior basketball season without any students allowed at games, but Peter was always upbeat and happy to be playing.

Finally football season arrived. It was quite cold since it was early spring in Buffalo instead of the usual late summer/early fall. Nobody had been more excited for Peter's senior football season than Zach. His absence was palpable. I had a hand towel made for Peter that read, *All for you Zach* with a #2 on it in honor of Zach, and Peter wore it in his back pocket for every game.

The first two games were so much fun. Peter was having a great senior season. It felt so good to be doing something "normal." Football had been part of our family routine for almost twenty years. At the same time, it hurt my heart that Zach wasn't with us. I knew without a doubt that he was there though, probably running next to Peter on every play yelling, "Yepp!!!!"

At one of the games, a friend of a friend came over to me and said that she didn't want me to think she was crazy, but she had something to tell me. She said that she is an intuitive and that she had a message for me from Zach: "Tell my mom I love her." She said that he wouldn't leave her alone until she came over to tell me. I laughed. Sounds about right.

The third game was Senior Night for football. Christopher came home for it. Peter and I walked our senior #1 out onto the field. Our hearts were all heavy. I look at the photos of all of us from that day and we are smiling but our eyes are sad. I can't imagine how Peter felt without Zach there for his games. He caught for over 100 yards that game and then I saw him go down and I knew he was badly hurt. He hobbled off the field. The team doctor had been our family pediatrician for 24 years and he looked at us and said, "Jen and Pete, get him to the hospital right away for X-rays. Don't wait." And so our whole family left the game and took Peter for X-rays where they found that he had broken his tibia.

He left on crutches. His senior year of football and his entire football career was over. Just like that. I couldn't believe it. Hadn't he been through enough??

True to form, Peter never complained. Not once. He went to every practice and every game for the rest of the season and cheered his teammates on, and there is no one more enthusiastic than Peter. (I still fondly remember when he played Little Loop, he would lead the team cheer before each game and his enthusiasm was contagious.) He was just as excited for his teammates scoring and playing well as if he were doing it himself. I've never been so proud of him. They went to the championship game, but lost. Peter told me that he cried because his teammates were crying. He is an empath; he could feel their sadness, but he has always had that innate understanding that it's just a game. He is a wise old soul.

As spring emerged, I felt a slight shift in my grief. I still cried every day, and I still missed Zach every day, but I wasn't in pain 24 hours a day anymore. As Jillian had suggested, I began to have some days when I wasn't focused on Zach's death every minute of the day.

I was starting to be able to find joy amid the sorrow. I had sadness and pain every day, but I was able to truly have some happy moments too. I was taking reiki clients again and I am sure that healing energy was helping me too. I continued to do daily breathing techniques, meditation and yoga. I continued to meditate and focus on Zach and feel his energy, his presence. It became easier to feel his presence all the time, not just when I meditated. I constantly asked him for signs and received signs. Life was still very hard.

At the end of April 2021, Kerry and I had another reading with Red. She had given me a reading for a Christmas gift and another for my birthday.

> Red: *On the physical plane, and the time with your son here on the physical plane, picture it as if his star is shining light through his body and your star is shining light through your body, but your stars are really right beside each other so those communications have happened for eternity anyway. So when his star no longer has a body to shine on, it doesn't take away the connection and the relationship that's there.*
>
> *So where you are, there is a sense of missing him because he's not there. But it's not like that for him because we are always here. It's a different experience for him. So all of the signs he does for you. He doesn't need to 'call home,' but you need him to 'call home.' He does that for you. If you're feeling down or low or missing him, he gives you a 'boost,' a sign to be supportive and to maintain a connection with the life that's going on without him; to have a presence in the life that's continuing without him.*

I ask about signs that he gives me. He verifies that Zach gives me cardinals and bluejays. "*Zach says, 'You can't influence elephants like that.'*" He is still making me laugh.

> Red: *He says the puppy sees his energy and you say, 'Hi Zach!' He has fun with it.*
>
> *He's not worried about being forgotten.*

You're still carrying the idea that if you had not taken your focus off him for a moment, this could have been averted, that he would be alive. That's not healthy for you. The worst has already happened and all of your vigilance wouldn't have changed that. You can't carry that responsibility.

You feel guilty because you didn't focus on him every moment when he was alive, and now you feel guilty when you're not focused on the pain all day. Recognize that life becomes centered around the pain less and less. And that is what should happen.

He didn't realize he was part of an epidemic. He knows that now.

He encourages his family to heal from this, because he doesn't want his legacy to be a legacy of pain.

Zach says he loves when his brothers are together. He just likes being in their energy. Especially when they're together and being rambunctious, he just likes being with them. He always did.

Zach says he really appreciates how Kerry stepped up and is looking after his mom.

I asked about how my boys were doing.

Red: *You tried to shield your grief from them and when you shared with them, they shared with you. You are all on the same journey. You let them know that everyone blames themself. Everyone secretly believes it was their fault. Do you know why people do that? Because it makes people think they have control over something that they have no control over. Nobody had control over it. Control is an illusion.*

The pain of losing Zach will always be there for all of you, but life will evolve around the pain.

He knows about the foundation you set up in his name. It makes him feel good that something might make a difference for those like him. He says, 'Thank you.' If he were alive he would be wiping his tears that he is being honored this way. He doesn't want his legacy to be of pain. You know that one, the last thing he would want is to inflict any pain on anyone. That's not the way of his soul. He knows that he caused the most pain possible to the ones he loves the most.

He knows now that there are many souls on that side that went through what he did. He is helping those on that side who crossed like he did.

He says, 'Don't worry about me anymore. I am good!'

All that's left is the love.

It was another reading that brought me so much comfort and even though I could hear Zach clearly sometimes, I couldn't hear him like that. It was like having a conversation with him and I think that these readings saved me sometimes. It was interesting that Zach said he hadn't realized that he was part of an epidemic. As his parents, it is important to us that people know that Zach wasn't just another overdose statistic; he was a beautiful soul.

It was so funny that Zach brought up his puppy interactions. I would often see Blue staring at the big photo of my boys behind me, specifically at Zach. Or sometimes, he would just stare into the air above me, as if he was looking at someone. I knew it was Zach. I always say, "Hi Zach!" and I love that Red acknowledged that.

In May, we had another significant event happen. I had received a call a few months prior from a woman at the University of Buffalo who told me that UB was awarding Zach a posthumous diploma because he was only a few credits away from graduating. I didn't even know that they did such a thing. Tears streamed down my face when she told me that Zach would would be graduating from UB. It's what he always wanted and always worked towards.

Our whole family was invited to the Dean's office for the ceremony. Our family plus Francine and Zach's Lily all went to receive Zach's diploma. I was overwhelmed with emotion when the Dean presented it to Peter and me. It was so bittersweet; bitter because we would rather have had Zach there to receive his diploma, but so sweet because he worked so hard for SO many years to earn it. I was so proud of him and I know that he was proud of himself too. He graduated magna cum laude, even with all of the obstacles he had faced while in school.

We all went out for dinner afterward and it was truly a celebration. Oh how I was wishing Zach was there. Just then, Kim and TJ Burch walked in. They were meeting friends at the next table. I told them what we were celebrating and we all laughed. Zach and Nolan brought in Nolan's parents for the celebration. Of course. It was a wonderful night.

Before we knew it, it was the end of Peter's senior year. He went to Senior Prom and we had a pre party at my house with four of his closest friends and their parents. They had been friends since middle school and their parents had become good friends of ours as well.

Because of Covid, his high school graduation ceremony took place at the Bills stadium since it was outside. It was very cool. We took the usual family photos after the ceremony. It was the first family milestone without Zach there. Peter's friend's family had a party afterward for everyone. We went out for a family graduation dinner a few days later. It was wonderful to celebrate and I was so proud of Peter, but my heart felt heavy. It felt so wrong that Zach wasn't there. I can't imagine how hard it was for Peter to graduate from high school without his big brother there.

It was a constant roller coaster of emotions for me. My "baby" was graduating from high school and soon going off to college, which is emotionally challenging for any mom, and then on top of it was the constant reminder that Zach wasn't there.

Since tenth grade, Peter had aspired to attend the University of Tampa in Florida. Since college applications were due right after Zach died, we were slightly late in getting them out and while he had been accepted to all of the colleges that he was interested in, he did not get into Tampa U for fall semester; he was accepted for spring semester 2022. I did make several phone calls to see if they could amend that, but UT had a record amount of applicants that year and there was nothing they could do. Part of me was relieved that he would stay in Buffalo for six more months. I worried that it was too soon for him to be away from his family, even though Christopher would be close by.

Peter would complete his first semester of college at SUNY Erie where Eric was going. Eric had gone to SUNY Erie for a year and then decided to take time off and work full time. He worked for a local company called Buffalo Strive Vending and he got up at 4:00 am every day for two years, bought a car, and banked a good amount of money. I was incredibly proud of his work ethic and how much he had matured. He then decided to return to school, while working part time. It was so nice that Eric and Peter were going together. They even had a class together.

CHAPTER TWENTY SEVEN

Summer came, the first summer without Zach. It was usually my favorite time of year. I love warm summer nights, sunsets, and being on or near the water when it's warm. It felt so sad to me doing anything fun without Zach here. As Red had said, I was struggling with the guilt of not being focused on the pain every minute. Sometimes I felt guilty feeling joy, even though I knew that's what Zach wants most, for us to feel joy.

Then one day Keith and I went for the first boat ride of the summer. Keith has a motorboat that he docks downtown and one of my favorite things to do in the summer is to spend an evening on the water. Our Buffalo sunsets are beautiful. My favorite thing is to stand at the front of the boat as it glides over the water, feeling the summer air hitting my face. On that first boat ride after Zach died, I was doing just that when I clearly heard Zach say, *"Now I know why you love this so much."*

He was there. He was with me. I could feel him and I clearly heard him and I knew that I didn't imagine it. Many times over the years we had invited Zach to come for a boat ride, but he never did. Peter loves boating and came out many times, including taking his friends tubing with us. Eric and Christopher had come out too, but never Zach. Now he is always with me on a boat ride. I was reminded once again that it is when I am feeling that joy from within, raising my vibration, that I can feel and hear Zach the clearest.

In June we had another reading. My dear friend Maria had gifted me her reading with Peggy Lynch, a gifted medium in Orchard Park that I had gone to several times after Peter's mom died. When I tried to set up the appointment with Peggy, she said that Zach told her that he wanted our whole family there for this one. Zach's dad declined and Christopher was in Tampa, so Eric, Peter, Kerry and Keith joined me for the reading. Some of the highlights from it were:

> Peggy: *When I come in with him, there is a feeling of serenity and peace. The addiction and mental illness left him as soon as he crossed. Zach wants you to know that he tried so hard.*

(Yes we know how hard he tried.)

> *His heart was really pure and IS pure. He is with a dog all the time. Did you get a new dog? This dog is a maniac, isn't he? Cray cray.*

(Peggy is hilarious. We all laugh. Yes he is.)

> *Zach is with him a lot. He really loves him and it's a connection between him and all of you. This dog will be a puppy for a long time.*

(She was right about that!)

She talks about Zach overdosing at Peter's house, that he went there deliberately to take the Opana, but that it wasn't an intentional overdose.

> *It was not suicide. He wants you to know that. He didn't want to break your hearts.*

> *He felt like his Aunt Kerry was like a big sister. He says he knew he could always go to her too. He loved his brothers.*

She talked about his OCD at length and how the drugs eased it.

> *Can you imagine how many hours a day he spent with his*

*OCD and yet still was a great student and an excellent ath-
lete.*

She talked about Morgan, a friend he had met at Sierra Tucson that he was very close to. He was worried about her.

She asked about a recent ceremony and when we said there was a ceremony for his posthumous diploma, she said that Zach was there. (Of course.)

She talked about the stuffed animal that was a gift for me. (Pluto dog.)

She referenced the last time that he was with all of us in a family situation. We realized it was Peter's birthday celebration at my house two days before he overdosed. She said that that's how he wants us to remember him, not how he was in the hospital.

> Peggy: *Zach says, ' Mom, you did everything you could.' He
> wants to reassure you of that. When you cross over, he will
> be there for you front and center over everybody. But you
> have a long life line. Because you have work to do. And you
> have to be here for your boys.*
>
> *Zach says that you don't have the patience with people that
> you used to and he says, 'It's about time, mom. I know you're
> protecting yourself and your heart and you really keep it
> tight with the family. But you always did.'*

She talked about a flower that popped up unexpectedly... on Mother's Day, at his grave.

(I remembered that when we went there for Mother's Day, I saw a blue carnation hanging from Zach's grave and I didn't know how it got there!)

She referenced the trip that Zach and I took together (NYC) and she said that Zach was really happy about the time we spent together. I had brought a scarf to the reading that I bought for Zach in NYC. When she held it, Zach said it was mom energy, and gave him the feeling of love and home.

She talked about Lily:

Peggy: *She was the one... if he hadn't had his struggles. He would have married her, if he wasn't so sick.*

She asked several times if Peter's wife Melissa has a child. We said no, but she has a dog. (Stay tuned for that one…)

Once again, having this reading was really healing and comforting for me. It also wasn't as heavy as they were in the beginning and Zach's humor was really coming through. Every reading made me feel close to him.

The Morgan that Peggy had referenced was a friend that Zach had met in treatment at ST and they were very close. She had reached out to me a few months after Zach died:

Hi Jennifer! First off, I miss your son all the time, he was one of the all time best and I was so lucky to have the relationship I had with him. Also, thanks for being the best mom anyone could ask for.

I was teaching a free yoga class at a place that I was working out of, and they had promoted that people could take the class on Instagram live. Morgan had seen the post and she and some others from ST had taken the class. Of course I just loved this. After that class, she began taking my weekly online Zoom yoga class from Colorado. The first time I saw her pretty face on the screen, I felt how happy Zach was that she was there. He obviously led her to the class.

A few months later, she texted:

Your Zach should have been healed. He deserved it more than anyone.

She said that she was trying to quit alcohol and that Zach always promoted that.

He was such a good healer down here but I keep telling myself that he is looking down healing me now too.

A couple months later, she told me that she had gone back to treatment and that she knew that Zach had led her there. She said that she has the best guardian angel. He gives her signs of 111, 11:11, and 444. She kept up with treatment and I am so happy to report that she is two years sober now and living a happy life.

That summer, another friend of Zach's from Sierra Tucson reached out to me. Her name is Jenny. Once again, because Zach's Instagram was open on my phone, I saw that she tagged him in a post and that is how we connected. It was Zach's doing, I am sure. She immediately shared her story with me of how Zach had saved her life, after he died. She met him at ST in February 2020. She wrote:

> I remember him telling his story and I was automatically drawn to him as I could relate to so much of his story and I was amazed and inspired by his strength, courage, resiliency, and not only his fight, but his want and willingness to fight and to be okay and to get better.

She said that after she had come home from ST, she was really struggling and knew in her heart she had to go back, but she was scared and felt stuck. She was suicidal, but felt like she couldn't make the decision on her own to go back to residential treatment because she felt so much shame (even though she knew it wasn't shameful at all). As she was struggling with making the decision, she kept seeing the numbers 111 and 11:11 (often referred to as angel numbers) after Zach died and then she kept seeing them more and more. (Zach gives me 11:11 as a sign as well.)

> Jenny: And then I knew with my whole heart that Zach was giving me a sign - so many signs! That it was ok to go back and he had been, and would continue to protect me so I could go back and get the help I need, so I could make the changes in my life that would allow me to live in recovery. I truly believe with my whole heart that he guided me back.

She calls him "her angel." When she booked her flight to go back to ST, the price was $111! When she got back to ST, she was sitting in a group counseling session and she was having a hard day and struggling and when she looked up, the chair in front of her had '*Call on an angel*' written on it. It was in the same building where she had met Zach for the first time. She knew Zach was giving her another sign. She said it was incredible. And after that, she never saw that chair again!

> Jenny: *If I didn't go back to ST, I would have lost my life to suicide and/or mental illness. I also struggle with OCD like Zach, and we have many similar struggles, and I know he understands what it's like and the pain that I was in. And through the angel numbers and signs that he has given me and continues to give me, I know that Zach saved my life. He is and forever will be so special, and I am continuing this fight for him because he was able to show me that it is worth it to continue fighting for myself as well.*

It was an incredible story for me to hear. When Zach died, we heard so many stories from people who said that he had saved their life. Now, I continue to hear stories about how he is saving lives from the other side. I am so proud of my Zach. That was two years ago. Since then, Jenny has completed inpatient, PHP, and then IOP and is now a recovery coach/case manager and peer supporter. We still stay in touch. I am so incredibly proud of her and I know that Zach is too.

When she was leaving ST, she painted a rock in honor of Zach to leave in the labyrinth there. She took a picture of it and sent it to me. We both noticed in the photo that there was a yellow name bracelet that was under Zach's rock. It said '*Jennifer M.*' I am Jennifer Marie. He is so clever.

The very same month, Raven, another one of Zach's friends from treatment, reached out to me through Facebook:

> *I would like to give my greatest condolences for your loss of Zach. I knew him from Huntington Creek, we would Face-Time often. It's nice to meet the mother of one of my greatest friends. I didn't reach out earlier because I was in my active addiction and I felt that would be disrespectful considering I only knew Zach sober, so I should give you the same respect.*

I want to say... Zach moving on... pushed me to realize I needed to better my life. He always had the biggest smile. I'd always tell him that his smile was the highlight of my morning.

So.. Zach is the reason I changed my life and moved to California. And... I just wanted to thank you for raising a wonderful young man.

I do it for Zach every day. And that's something that gives me strength and pushes me to do even more and more good with my life. Because now I'm trying not just for me, but for him too. That man had so much love to give the world, and I'm guessing he got that from you. Keep your head up. Much love and blessings.

Another friend of Zach's overdosed that summer and he said that Zach was with him when he was revived and Zach told him that it wasn't his time yet. He told me, '*Something genuinely flipped in that moment for me.. he saved my life.. not just in that moment but from everything we went through together here. Being sober since that day isn't a coincidence, I wouldn't be able to put a day together without him.*' He is now over two years sober.

There were more stories like these. I was truly overwhelmed with such gratitude for Zach helping all of these young people, and that they are all alive and doing well, but also utterly devastated that it couldn't be Zach who was alive and well. Still, it makes my heart happy to see their posts of how wonderfully they are all doing. I am so proud of each and every one of them and most of them I have never even met. It makes me feel close to Zach whenever they reach out to me.

Even though I was doing better than I had been nine months earlier, some days were still a struggle to get through. I struggled with the unfairness of it all. Peter and I both struggled with the fact that there are heroin and meth addicts who lived on the street for many years and they are alive. Why couldn't that be Zach? Of course I am happy for all of the addicts who got to live, of course I am. I would never wish this nightmare on any parent. But why couldn't Zach have lived? We never thought that Zach had deliberately overdosed; we knew he wanted to get better and have a happy life, and several of the mediums addressed that Zach wanted us to know that. Several of them also mentioned that there was fentanyl in the drug that killed him. I have always suspected that as well, but we didn't have it tested. He was gone.

Some of the moms I knew were planning showers, weddings, and baby showers for their kids, while I had just planned a funeral for my son. I was "stuck" in the unfairness of life.

As luck would have it, Jillian began a monthly "check in" with those of us who have been working with her for years. These check in's were such a blessing to me. Each month she would help me with spiritual counseling and give me a particular meditation to do for the month.

That summer, I texted her how I was feeling:

> Some days I feel like I'm going backwards. It's hard not to ask, 'Why did my 24 year old son have to die? Why is life SO hard?'

She called me. She reminded me that she is usually a "tough love" kind of teacher and that what she was about to say may seem harsh. She said, "If it FEELS good to you to think, 'Why did my 24 year old son have to die?,' then stick with that. OR… if it feels better in your heart to say, 'I am so grateful for the 24 years I got to spend with Zach on earth and for the love and close bond that we shared. And I am so grateful for the continued love and bond that we share with him on the other side.' If that feels better in your heart, then go with that one. And if I were you, I'd want to punch me right now."

(She is a funny one.)

She was right of course. It didn't make me feel good to think that way. And it certainly didn't help anyone around me. And it certainly didn't make Zach happy. I had been working on controlling my thoughts for years. I know that our thoughts literally create our world. However as we all know, it is harder than it seems. Still, I needed Jillian's tough love to push me forward with my healing. If I couldn't get out of my own head, I knew that I would have an unhappy life without Zach here. That's not what he wants and that is not what my boys want.

So when I notice my thoughts going down that dark path, I use what Jillian said as my mantra, "*I'm so grateful that I got to spend 24 years with my Zach and for the bond we shared and still share. I'm so grateful that he's always with me.*" Three years later, I still have those moments and I still go back to that mantra. I close my eyes and take a deep breath and I feel my Zach with me. It helps tremendously.

That summer my sister Kerry went to a psychic medium named Leanne while she was on vacation with a friend. Zach was waiting for her. She spoke at length about how he suffered with mental illness and only used the drugs to quiet his mind.

> Leanne: *He says that he never wanted to hurt his family. He's sorry he hurt his mom. He knows it almost broke her. He loves her.*

She said he was showing her Led Zeppelin, ZZ Top, something with a Z. Kerry laughed and said that his name is Zach and that he gives her Led Zeppelin and ZZ Top for signs.

She said that Zach kept saying he is with the little girl in the family, with the chocolate brown hair and that he will always be with her. Kerry said that there is no little girl in the family. Zach kept talking about the little girl, so finally Leanne spoke into Kerry's phone which was recording the reading, '*This is a message to Zach's family: just know that Zach is going to take care of the little girl with the chocolate brown hair in this family.*'

We thought it was odd. A week later, Peter and Melissa told me that they were having a baby. She was 12 weeks pregnant. They had gotten married six months after Zach died. I was happy for both of them, but I was especially happy that Peter would have a baby to help heal his broken heart. Kerry and I knew that this was the little girl that Zach had been talking about.

After that, it became a regular occurrence for Zach to crash other people's readings with mediums. Eric's friend Angie had a reading and he showed up with a message for Eric. My friend Annmarie had a reading to try and connect with a dear friend who had just passed, and Zach showed up and basically hijacked the reading with beautiful messages for me. One day, a mom I knew from Wanakah contacted me and said, "You're not going to believe this...." And I said, "Oh I will believe it!" She lived out of state but Zach still crashed her reading to give messages to me.

Because Kerry's reading with Leanne had been so amazing, I then did a phone reading with her myself.

> Leanne: *Do you know how much he loved you? He was a good boy. He feels at peace now. He is with his grandma. He is with Bailey. He tried hard not to use.*
>
> *People loved him. He didn't even know how many people loved him.*
>
> *He gives you bluejays and 11:11.*
>
> *You were so close to him. And he's so sorry he pulled away at the end and didn't tell you everything.*
>
> *He was kind to everyone. He was good to everyone that he touched.*
>
> *He said to tell Lily that she tried to save him a couple of times, but he did what he wanted to do. He said to tell her not to feel guilty.*

She asked about a sports team that his dad would be watching on tv. I laughed and said, "The Bills. A football team." She said to tell his dad that Zach watches the games with him and he follows him around.

(This is funny because Peter paces around nervously, walking in and out of the house during Bills games.)

Leanne: *He loves Francine and knows she is taking it hard.*

He wants you to stay on earth. You have to live for him.

He wants his brothers to love each other and he wants to be an uncle someday.

He loves the new puppy.

She said that Zach is loud as Hell. Too funny. Yepp. All the mediums say that he is loud and clear.

CHAPTER TWENTY EIGHT

A COUPLE MONTHS AFTER Zach died, Peter and I had set up the foundation in his memory. We wanted the money that Jonathan had raised at the Wanakah dinner to be put immediately into a foundation, even if we had no idea where we were donating it yet. When choosing a name for the foundation, we considered variations on Zach's initials, but we were in agreement; it would be named the Zach Liberatore Foundation. Simple, in memory of our Zach.

My Sue was the first person to ask to be on our board of directors and we were honored. We knew that we wanted to have a fundraiser and we talked about it being in October, to mark the year anniversary of Zach's death, but it seemed like a daunting task and we were still in deep grief. My inspiration for all of this were the Burch's, Nolan's parents. Kim and TJ had started the NMB Foundation after Nolan died, to spread awareness of the dangers of hazing. For eight years, they have travelled all over the country, lecturing to high school and college students and talking about their son's death. There was a documentary made by their friend Dan Catullo, along with WVU, called "Breathe, Nolan, Breathe" which follows the events that unfolded when Nolan overdosed on alcohol and passed. It has won many awards, including an Emmy award. Courageous is the only word I can use to describe Kim and TJ for showing that documentary over and over with the sole purpose of saving lives. I am very sure that they have.

That summer, Sue began to gently pressure us. She suggested that she could set up a coffee date with some women that she knew who were all knowledgeable about foundations/fundraising and who wanted to help. Even though we were excited about the foundation, it sounded exhausting. Finally we had no choice; Sue set up a date at the end of summer for Peter, Melissa and I to meet with Sue and her friends. We had no idea what to expect. I honestly thought that they would give us some advice and that we would have our first fundraiser with pizza and sell tickets at the door. We had no idea what was coming. These women (I call them our angels) descended on us with a whirlwind of questions and ideas. What was our mission? When will the first fundraiser be? What is our logo? Do we have a website? Who would be the "face" of the foundation? (Besides Zach of course.) We spent two hours with them describing our mission and brainstorming ideas for a fundraiser in October. That gave us less than two months to find a venue and all that goes with that, set up a committee, set up a website, and start marketing the event. We were shocked that they all wanted to be on the event committee and help.

Linda had many years of experience hosting events. Theresa was in marketing. Colleen was an attorney with experience on boards. Maureen was an accountant who would help with the money aspect. And of course my Sue, who is extremely successful in business. We came up with various ideas for venues to check for availability. I thought that we would have a couple hundred people, but they were all sure that we would need a bigger space for more people than that.

We decided that we needed a logo immediately. We had tossed around ideas with a football, but then Peter said, "Z. It has to be just Z. Because he was Z." Yes. Everyone called him Z. I said, "Yes! But it's missing something." Melissa was sitting next to me and then it was as if someone pushed my head down and I was looking at the tattoo on her wrist that she had gotten for Zach. It was a Z with a semicolon. Z; "That's it!" I said. I was giddy.

That's exactly what Zach would want and I am sure that he was the one who brought it to my attention.

In mental health, the semicolon tattoo began as a symbol of someone who had attempted suicide, but lived. Now the semicolon has come to symbolize solidarity against depression, addiction, and mental illness; continuing your story. Zach always wanted to get a semicolon tattoo, but his OCD wouldn't allow it. This was the perfect symbol for Zach. His story isn't over. We will continue to tell his story and we will continue to be an advocate for mental health, the way he was.

Our heads were spinning after that meeting. There was so much to do. Sue and I stayed after the meeting to process and talk. A few minutes later, Melissa texted me:

We could call the fundraiser Zachtoberfest.

Oh my gosh! That was perfect! Just then, the barista yelled out, "Order for Zachary!" Sue and I looked at each other and laughed. Zach liked that idea.

The next two months were a whirlwind. It was as if the whole thing took on a life of it's own and we were dragged along with it. Peter and I knew that before we started to advertise the event, we wanted to determine where these funds would be donated. People would want to know where their donations were going. Obviously Zach struggled with addiction, so we could choose a recovery program to donate to. When we were planning his services, we asked that instead of people sending flowers (even though I love flowers), they donate to Save the Michaels of the World, an organization in Buffalo which provides awareness and support for drug addiction. However, Peter and I were in agreement that Zach would want this money raised to go towards helping kids and young people with OCD in Western New York. We had no idea how since there was no OCD outpatient clinic here. I always say that Zach died of an overdose, but it wasn't addiction that killed him; it was his severe, debilitating OCD that plagued him for eight years. If he didn't have the OCD, he wouldn't have had addiction.

I called Chris, Zach's last psychologist to ask if he had a suggestion. He said that actually, Oishei Children's Hospital of Buffalo had started an OCD Clinic before Covid, but then it had to be shut down. It would be the first OCD Outpatient Clinic in Buffalo. He said he would pass the information along to Dr. Benedict, who was the manager of the Child Psychiatric Clinic. Dr. Benedict called me and said that this was divine intervention. The program could not move forward without funding. I think we were both crying. Divine intervention and Zach intervention I'm sure. Everything was falling into place perfectly.

Our committee grew rapidly and each person brought something unique to the table. Peter's cousin Michelle came on board, who has been planning events for her family's company her whole life. Melissa's friend Adele offered to lead our basket raffle. She had lost her Zack to addiction as well. And Melissa herself is a real estate agent who is great at marketing. My friend Wendy offered to lead our silent auction, even though she runs her own fundraiser at her job. Her son Connor was a longtime friend of Zach. Of course our Francine came on board who always has great ideas. Michelle's friend DJ Anthony volunteered to donate his time and music. There is no doubt that Zach had a hand in all of this. I know that he brought all of these incredible people to us.

Next we needed to create a website. Peter had a friend at Medaille College who said he would meet with us. We obviously wanted to keep costs low. He immediately said, "I think we should bring Hannah Taylor in." Hannah. Another angel sent to us. I connected with her instantly; she is spiritual and intuitive and a healer as well. She was compassionate and empathetic to our story and said she would do anything to help. She said that I could send her all of the text, as well as photos, and she would design our website.

That day, I emailed Hannah everything that I wanted on our website. I wrote Zach's "story." Theresa had put together our official "Mission statement." Peter's cousin Mary, who is in graphic design, graciously created our Z; logo based on Melissa's tattoo. Most importantly to me, I wanted Zach's essay on our website that truly sheds light on what severe OCD really is. We needed a main photo of Zach and a color scheme.

After Zach died, his friend Troy sent me a recent picture that he had taken. It was a beautiful photo of my Zach. It was perfect for the website and posters. I have a blown up copy of it hanging in my kitchen. One day, I was sitting at my kitchen table trying to figure out what our color scheme would be. We had been toying with the idea of Bills colors: red, blue and white. I was looking at the photo of Zach and then I knew. His shirt in that photo is royal blue and black. That was it. UB colors. Zach was directing me every step of the way.

I sent all of that information to Hannah and by the time I woke up the very next morning, she had sent me a link to our Zach Liberatore Foundation website. It was so beautiful, so perfect that I cried when I saw it. She had used every photo I had given her and placed them throughout the website. Hannah had taken our vision and made it even more beautiful than I could have imagined. I was so incredibly grateful.

Hannah has continued to help us with updates to our website over the years, as well as other media design. (She is also a talented artist and created the beautiful cover design for this book.)

The way that our family and friends and community stepped up to support our fundraiser still gives me chills. People donated money, baskets for the basket raffle and amazing silent auction items. We even had a Bills helmet signed by Josh Allen! (I know Zach loved that.) Sue is our volunteer coordinator and we had over 50 people volunteer to work the event. Sue's entire family, the Walsh's, were volunteers. All of the Liberatore cousins volunteered. And my friend Lillian had recruited a team of Orchard Park moms.

As Zachtoberfest approached, October 2nd came upon us, the one year anniversary of Zach's death. It was heart wrenching. More than anything, I couldn't believe that it had been a year since I saw his face, since I hugged him. I went to the cemetery alone. It was such a difficult day and my heart felt so heavy. Then our family went out for dinner: my boys, Peter, Melissa, my sister, Peter's sister, Francine and Lily. Instead of it being a depressing evening, it was actually fun and we laughed a lot. It was Francine's birthday.

I hadn't realized at the time that Zach had died on her birthday. Recently I read a story about a mom who was devastated because her son had committed suicide on her birthday. She found out in a reading that he did that so that she would always remember him. Perhaps that's what Zach did for Francine, one of his favorite people. After dinner, we drove to the waterfront to release Chinese lanterns in the dark. We had to keep relocating because the wind was blowing the lanterns towards the boats. Peter said Zach was messing with us. No doubt. I think he was trying to prolong the evening. The boys were playing music and dancing and I know that Zach was right in the middle of them. We were blessed to make it through that day feeling some joy along with the sorrow.

Before we knew it, the day arrived of our first annual Zachtoberfest. I don't think I've ever been so nervous for an event before. We had the best team imaginable but at the end of the day, it was our foundation and if it didn't go well, we would feel terrible. We worried about the food, if the payment squares didn't work, or if we didn't have enough volunteers to handle everything. It was all new.

We worked all day setting up. We had an astounding 109 baskets and over 50 silent auction items. It was a daunting task. Oishei Children's Hospital (OCH) had linked us with someone from their foundation (Melissa) and she became an instant friend. Melissa had all of our signs made through OCH and I had tears in my eyes when I walked around before the event began. "Z," was everywhere in "Zach blue." All of the volunteers wore "Z," t-shirts. The photo slide show set to music that I had made for the wake ran all night on all of the screens. We all had tears in our eyes when it started to play.

I had injured my knee that week, so I stood at the top of the stairs leading into the event since it hurt to walk. The rest of our family was all over talking to people, but I ended up standing in that spot all night as people kept streaming in. It was really unbelievable. I was completely overwhelmed by the amount of people who came to support our family and honor our Zach. It turned out to be over 800 people in attendance and it was a room filled with love. Our good friend Dennis said to me, "When I die, there will not be this many people. This is all for Zach. Everyone loved Zach." I laughed. Everyone did love Zach.

Dr. Jennifer Haak, one of the OCH psychiatrists, spoke about what OCD really is and how debilitating it can be. Many people told me that her speech was very enlightening. I spoke as well, even though I was extremely nervous, thanking our committee, volunteers, and everyone who supported us.

It was truly a magical night. Christopher said that he felt like he "slapped up" every person that he has ever known. We were all overwhelmed with gratitude. I could feel Zach all night. Of course. More than anything, it was fun. I wasn't even remotely concerned about how much money we raised, but we were shocked to find out that we had raised $100,000 that night, all thanks to our generous community. It was truly unbelievable. After paying out for costs, food and venue, we were so blessed to be able to present a check for $85,000 to Oishei Children's Hospital's Psychiatric Clinic and OCD Program. Zach was so proud.

At one point during the evening, I was taking a video of the sea of faces, and I suddenly remembered what Jillian had told me a year ago almost to that exact day: "You won't believe the amazing thing that you and Zach will accomplish a year from now. You won't believe it." Yes - Zach, me, Peter, Melissa, Sue, Michelle, and our entire committee. Simply amazing. We kept our promise to Zach to keep his name alive and to continue his compassionate legacy of helping people. I am forever indebted to our family, our friends, and our community for making it all possible. What I remember most is seeing all of my boys happy. Once again, their friends had come from all over to support them and honor Zach. That night, our foundation was able to bring meaning and purpose into our lives. It has helped us heal, and continues to do so. I am eternally grateful for that.

CHAPTER TWENTY NINE

Sue's sister Maggi said to me at Zachtoberfest, "Look around and take it all in. Don't do anything tomorrow besides feeling the joy of accomplishment." Oh, if only that were possible.

The very next day, my sister Kerry and I found ourselves in another nightmare. Our dad had been diagnosed with throat cancer prior to Zachtoberfest. He had just had a scope and his health was deteriorating rapidly, aggravated by the scope. He was our mom's primary caregiver. Our mom had many health problems and was basically bound to a wheelchair at this point, unable to climb the stairs. We all knew that my mom needed to be placed in a full care facility, but dad had been refusing, until now.

Now he could barely take care of himself. I began the daunting task of calling nursing homes. After Covid, there were few or no beds available anywhere. Also, my mom had been in and out of nursing homes for years for rehab and we were not happy with some of them. She would have to leave their home to live in a nursing home for the rest of her life; I felt the weight of the world on my shoulders to get her into an excellent facility. I also hoped that it could be close by so that my dad could easily get to see her. I remember standing in their family room, staring at a photo of Zach. I'd only lost him a year ago. I didn't know how much more I could take.

We ended up having to take my mom to Mercy Hospital, the hospital where Zach had died. I had hoped I would never have to walk into that hospital ever again. When we were in the ER with her, I forced myself to walk over to the room where the ER doctor had told us that Zach had died in the ambulance. It all came back and I stood there and sobbed while doctors and nurses looked at me with pity.

My mom was admitted to the hospital, but if she was not accepted into one of the nursing homes we had applied to, she could be sent anywhere. I was trying to get her into a place in Orchard Park that had excellent reviews and my dad and I had checked out years before. The nurse suggested that I call the hospital social worker and then by some miracle, she happened to be on that floor.

She came in and when I introduced myself, she asked if I was related to Delaney (Zach's cousin) who was her daughter's best friend. Yes! Zach had been very close to Delaney and her daughter! I said that I was Zach's mom and we all cried. I told her our predicament and she said that she knew someone at the nursing home we were hoping to get into, and she would make a call for us. The next morning, during my dad's surgery, I got a text from her that my mom had been accepted there and could go immediately. It was a huge weight off of my shoulders. Clearly Zach had orchestrated this, sending in his friend's mom to so kindly help us. I knew without a doubt that Zach was right by my side, helping me.

For the next two months, Kerry and I moved our mom into the nursing home and took turns taking our dad to Roswell Park Cancer Institute for doctor's appointments and radiation treatments. He had stage four throat cancer and his decline was quick and aggressive. It was heartbreaking to see our dad like this. He wasn't even strong enough to visit mom. We took him and my boys to see mom on Christmas and cried as our mom and dad hugged. We all knew that it was probably the last time they would see each other.

On New Year's Eve, my mom was rushed back to Mercy Hopital with MRSA pneumonia. The next morning, on New Year's Day, my dad called us to call an ambulance for him. As the paramedics wheeled him away, he winked at us. He knew. We took turns staying with each of our parents on different floors of the hospital. Late that night, we went home and then got a call that dad was code blue. We rushed back to the hospital, but it was too late. Dad had crossed over. The paramedic team who had cared for him was very kind to us. The young man said his name was Zach. His name tag said, "Zachary." Another sign. At the time that my dad passed, I was driving and I had a clear vision of Zach taking my dad by the hand. Of course I knew they were together. I was envious.

The nurses were all so compassionate and empathetic to our situation. We told them that my Zach had died there a year ago. We told them that our mom was on the next floor and we had to go and tell her that her husband was gone. They said they had never heard such a sad story. I was hanging on by a thread. We went up and told my mom. They had been married for 59 years. He was her other half. She was not well and it didn't look like she was going to make it. It all felt like a bad dream.

No matter how old you are, it is difficult to lose a parent. After losing my 24 year old son, it was obviously a different kind of grief to lose my 84 year old dad who had a good, long life. But my dad was my rock. My hero. There is a special bond between a girl and her dad. For my sister, our dad was the closest person to her in this life. We were relieved that he wasn't suffering anymore, but it was another big loss after just losing Zach. I believe that PTSD set in again. I pushed the grief down in order to take care of all of the tasks at hand. Mourning would come much later.

Our mom was actually slowly improving, but she was still in the hospital and wanted us to go ahead with the services, so we planned another wake and funeral. My brother Peter came in from Texas. I wrote another eulogy. It was surreal.

Two days later, we took Peter to Tampa and moved him into his dorm at University of Tampa. It was also my birthday. As we walked around the campus, I could see why Peter wanted to go there. We had a fun couple of days, shopping for his dorm room and all of us going out for dinners. It was therapeutic for me.

After our last dinner, I drove him back to his dorm and got out of the car to say goodbye. Peter has always had this innate understanding of things; he knew I would be emotional and he smiled knowingly, in complete understanding of how hard this was for me. I felt like my heart was breaking, leaving him there so far away from home, but I tried not to show it. It was a lot for me to handle so soon after Zach died, however I was so happy for him that he was moving forward with his plans and his life after losing his big brother. I was incredibly proud of his strength and maturity. Peter and I have always wanted to give our sons both roots and wings; to know they always have family and home to ground them and to know that they can "fly" and accomplish anything they set their minds to. Peter was doing just that, even after the trauma that we had just endured.

The next task was for Kerry and I to clean out our parents' house and put it on the market. They had 50 years worth of stuff; it was an overwhelming job ahead of us. It took us 15 weekends to clean it out and spruce it up. It was extremely emotional for us after losing our dad to get rid of all of his belongings and the home that he was so proud of. Slowly I let the mourning process begin. I believe that allowing myself to grieve the loss of my dad also brought up grief over Zach and that it helped me to heal.

Then another tragedy struck. Ryan Downing who had sung *Home* at Zach's funeral, died of an overdose. My heart broke for his parents and siblings. I went to the wake and hugged Angela tight and attended the funeral. It was too much for me only 16 months after Zach had died. It was difficult for me to keep it together, especially when I saw the raw, familiar pain on Angela's face. Ryan was a beautiful soul with the voice of an angel. I had no doubt that Zach was there for him when he crossed over.

Kerry had gotten me another Red reading for my birthday and we thought it was a good time to use it.

Red: *When your dad crossed over, Zach gave you a full image of him taking your dad by the hand. 'Come on grandpa! I've got things to show you!'*

(Oh my gosh he did! I thought that I envisioned that, but Zach was showing me.)

> Red: *Your connection with Zach is very clear, isn't it? You notice his responses are fast. He's proud of himself on his cross dimension connection. He says it's like he is carrying his cosmic cellular phone. He's a funny guy, isn't he?*

(Haha Yepp!)

> Red: *He says, 'This guy knows his stuff. There's a lot of me to go around now.'*
>
> *You ask him to do things for you, don't you Jennifer?*

(I say, "Yes I do! I'm probably annoying.")

> Red: *It's not annoying at all. There is no such thing as time where he is, so he can be everywhere at once.*
>
> *He says that his name now has a legacy. That is a gift that you all gave him. That's a joy for him. You brought the phoenix out of the ashes, based on who you knew he was.*
>
> *He feels that his story can help other people. He knows that it is many other people's story as well. He is helping people on that side, just like you are helping people there.*
>
> *He is sorry that he hurt everyone so bad. He would never want to hurt anyone. That was not his way.*
>
> *He knows that you still wrestle with the idea of 'How could I have helped more?'*
>
> *You knew that he was in pain, but he told you he was okay. You couldn't see what he didn't want you to see. It's important for you not to carry the blame because it causes anguish inside of you. He really wanted to handle it himself. He says, 'I'm okay now. You need to be okay. You didn't fail me. Nobody did.'*

*He knows that each lifetime is a blink. And it's a loving uni-
verse. He is having fun making things happen. What's left is
that pure line of love. Love and familiarity is the main line
of your connection.*

Zach knew that I was still struggling with, "How could I have helped
more? Why couldn't we save him?" This reading really helped me to solid-
ify in my mind the truth that I couldn't have done any more to help him. I
had heard that for years, and I knew in my heart it was true, but my mind
sometimes got the best of me.

I began to feel a shift in my grief, in my whole perspective. It finally hit
me that after all those years of asking God to heal Zach, God DID heal
Zach. Of course it wasn't healing him on earth the way I wanted it to be; it
was a more complete and perfect healing. He is now in the dimension of
pure love, Heaven, if that's what you call it. I call it "Home."

And what about the faith that I had my entire life… *Everything happens
for a reason.* Now that a tragedy had happened and my world had been
destroyed, I didn't believe that anymore?? No. I DID still believe it in my
heart. It just took awhile for my mind to catch up.

The fact is, I have always had very deep faith in God (or whatever you
choose to call the divine source that we all come from). I no longer align
with any organized religion because the judgment of others who follow a
different religion doesn't resonate with me. Please note that I am not criticizing any religion; I just haven't found one that fits. I still love to sit in
churches though, especially churches filled with angels.

The truth is, nothing makes us question our faith more than the loss of
the ones we love the most. It's easy to have faith when everything is easy
and going well. It was easy for me to have faith when all of my children
were alive. When Zach died, *Everything happens for a reason* seemed inherently wrong. I'm not supposed to bury my child. Yet, I finally had to accept
the fact that the faith that I had before Zach died hadn't changed.

Jillian always said, "Everything is exactly the way it is supposed to be. Or
it wouldn't be." And so, the only perspective on all of this was that Zach was

supposed to die. Or he wouldn't have. Whether he died of a drug overdose, or terminal cancer, or a fatal car accident, it would have happened somehow. Because it was supposed to. The saying, "Let go and let God" took on a whole deeper meaning. I knew that I had to let go.

Jillian had said that our souls chose this before we came into this life: Zach's, mine, and all of us. We all had to agree to it. I had heard the words, but it didn't really sink in until now. Clearly Zach was doing incredible work on the other side, and because of his death, we are doing work through his foundation to help children and young people here. Perhaps that is the "reason" for his death. We may never know. The truth is, it felt freeing to let go of all the other chatter in my head of "Why? Why? WHY?" and "Not fair!" All of that made me feel worse, not better. It felt better in my heart to reframe it to "Everything is exactly as it is supposed to be. Or it wouldn't be." It just felt better.

I'm not sure why after years of spiritual searching, lessons, books, readings, and counseling, it finally started to sink in, but it did. Perhaps it was because of the depth of the loss. The great poet Rumi said, *The wound is the place where the light enters you.* This I now comprehend on the deepest level, on a soul level.

We feel and hold grief in our heart chakra. Whenever I did, and still do, yoga poses for the heart chakra such as camel pose and bridge pose, I picture white light coming into the center of my chest and I speak a mantra to myself, *I allow the light to come in.* Over time, the combination of that physical practice plus the reframing of my thoughts of how I viewed Zach's crossing over, slowly healed my heart.

This is not to say that I wasn't still having painful moments or sadness, but I felt myself coming out of that all encompassing darkness and into the light. I wasn't having day after day of heavy grief anymore, in fact not even whole days of heavy grief. When I had moments of sadness, I allowed myself to feel it but instead of getting stuck in that sadness, I tried to move through it with a breathing technique or mantra.

Honestly I think that more than anything, it was about letting go of trying to control the outcome; letting go of thinking that we have control over what happens to our loved ones. For those of us who have lost a child, the biggest test is trying to come to terms with that. We don't have control over anything. Control is an illusion. The only thing that we can control is how we respond to what happens to us. There is a higher power in control and it does not matter what you call that higher power: Source, the Divine, Allah, the Universe, God … it is the pure love that we all came from and where we are all going back to. When I began to "let go," I felt a sense of calm and peace that I hadn't felt since long before Zach died. I also had to let go of the grief that I was clinging to so fiercely. I think that sometimes we cling to the grief as if it is our only connection to our loved one. Deep inside, I had been afraid that if I let go of that grief, what would be left? What's left is the love, and two souls that will always be together.

CHAPTER THIRTY

T HAT SPRING, WE finally had happy and exciting things happening. After all of the work that Kerry and I had done on our parents' house, it sold quickly with Melissa's help. It felt freeing to get that project finished.

Even more importantly, Peter and Melissa's baby was born. Truth be told, I harbored a secret fear that it would be a boy who looked like Zach and that would have tugged at my heartstrings, but of course it was a girl, just as the medium had suggested; Zach said he would always watch over the little girl with the chocolate brown hair. She was here.

Camellia Mary Liberatore was born that spring and she has brought nothing but joy into all of our lives ever since. All babies are a blessing, but she truly brought healing to our whole family. It was heartwarming to see Peter with her; he looked truly happy for the first time since Zach died. She adores all of her brothers, but she and Eric have a special bond because he sees her the most. They share blueberries together.

She is always happy and laughing and I am very sure that's because Zach is always with her and he's making her laugh. It is said that babies can easily see angels and souls from the other side because they are still "of that world." Sadly, most of them grow up and become jaded by the human perspective. Of course she is smiling all the time when she can see Zach's beautiful face smiling at her! I get to see her often as well. I find any excuse to stop over at their house to see her cute face.

It may sound absolutely crazy, but another thing that brought more joy into my life was the purchase of my Peloton bike. I had been going to spinning classes for 20 years, but then finally let go of my gym membership because it is easier to work out at home. I practice yoga, I use free weights, and I have a pilates reformer at home. That, plus running outside was my exercise routine. When running began to cause endless problems with my joints, I switched to walking, but I missed that cardio endorphin rush. I had multiple pieces of pilates equipment from when I was a studio owner, so I sold one of my reformers and bought the Peloton bike. It is one of the best purchases I have ever made.

While all of the Peloton instructors are awesome, a friend told me that Cody Rigsby is her favorite because he makes her laugh and I was sold. He makes me laugh out loud every time, whether he is doing a dissertation on toaster strudel, calling us dumdums for saying "expresso" instead of "espresso," or defending Ursula, the villain in *Little Mermaid*. (She isn't a villain, she is just a smart business woman.) We have the same taste in female singers, we both know that Whitney Houston was the GOAT, we are both ex-dancers, and when Cody Rigsby is dancing on the bike, so am I. I am grateful to him for making this broken hearted mama bear dance and laugh every morning.

I believe that also reminded me of the joy that dancing brings to me. On days when my grief took over, I would play one of my favorite feel good songs and dance by myself. That immediately raises my vibration. While dancing may not be the thing that brings you joy, I challenge you to dance and feel sad at the same time. It is almost impossible.

In May of 2022, I began writing this book. I have always known that I would write a book at some point in my life. I attribute this to my sixth grade teacher Mrs. Davis. She was a strict, no nonsense kind of teacher, so when she wrote on a short story that I wrote, "Remember me when you're a published author," I have believed ever since then that I would write a book. I had no idea what it would be about, but that shows what a powerful influence a teacher can have on a child. She put that idea in my head.

Zach was a beautiful and gifted writer. We both always knew that he would write a book someday. Eventually, I thought that we would write that book together, when he was better and had overcome all that he had gone through. After he died, I realized that we would still write a book together, except with him on the other side... my talented "ghost writer." Whenever I am writing, I ask him to co-write with me and I know that he does.

It was so much more difficult than I could have imagined. Even as I wrote about Zach's happy times as a child, it hurt my heart remembering the hopes and dreams that I had for him. It hurt too much. I took a break from it.

Soon after that, Keith and I attended an event at Shea's Performing Arts Center in Buffalo, where Renee Elise Goldsberry was performing. She is an incredibly talented broadway star. Between songs, she told a story about a friend of hers who had battled cancer and survived. That friend now helps others who are going through what she did. I swear that Renee Elise Goldsberry was looking directly at me when she said that it takes a courageous person who makes it through the tunnel of darkness to the other side, and then chooses to go back into the tunnel to help others through to the other side. Tears streamed down my face. I don't know if she told that story at every performance, but I knew that message was for me. Did I mention that she used to play Nala in *The Lion King* on Broadway? And so I got back to the writing of this book.

That summer, Kerry and I had yet another reading with Red:

> Red: *Zach recognizes and appreciates that his family is handling this with grace. He sees others who died in the same way, witness the suffering of their families. Some of these families are angry and ashamed and some of those people go into the deepest pits of despair and refuse to come out. He sees these struggles and he feels very blessed. He sees his*

family working to handle their grief and he so appreciates how you all are carrying this. He is really appreciative.

I ask if Zach has anything to say about the book.

Red: *You know when you start writing something and he corrects you. You start writing, and then you change it.*
Yes. I feel that.

Red talks about our foundation:

Red: *Everyone wants a happy ending, but in these types of stories, there isn't a happy ending. Everyone wants to resolve it. And you can't. It doesn't resolve. But you all took the tragedy of not having this bright soul there and you turned it into everything good that you can do.*

Zach wants it to be a foundation of hope. He wants you to focus on finding hope and building hope, based on the faith that kindness and compassion will prevail. He tried in his life to live as a kind and compassionate person. He tried to be inspiring to others in his life.

Yes he certainly did. He tried, and he succeeded.

It's interesting that while Zach's death could have impacted our family dynamic in a negative way, it instead has brought us all closer together. Because of Zach's foundation and all of the work that goes into the fundraisers, we all spend a lot of time together. In year two, we added to our committee: my sister, our friend Cheryl, and Melissa's assistant Trish. This year, our son Eric and Peter's sister Carol have also jumped on board.

We added a golf tournament to our docket that year as well, which Peter really wanted to do. His friend Ron and his cousin Michelle completely run it for him. It is a much smaller event than Zachtoberfest with 100 golfers, but Peter and our boys golf together and we all volunteer. It is always an uplifting and fun day, honoring our Zach.

Our committee meetings began that summer in preparation for our second annual Zachtoberfest. There is so much work involved for this fundraiser and we would be lost without each of the amazing women on our committee. They all have full time jobs and families, yet they fully commit to our event for the simple reason that they want to help. We are forever grateful to each of them for their commitment and expertise. I always say that if it were just Peter and me running this fundraiser, it would look very different.

Just in time for Zachtoberfest, my friend Renee finished a project we had been working on... a "Z" ring. I had the idea to take an old necklace that Peter had given me many years ago and make it into a ring with a diamond Z. Renee owns a jewelry store and we had been working on the design for a year. Her partner in the store was her brother and best friend, Kenny, who had died tragically years before. When Peter and I were picking out a burial place for Zach, I immediately noticed that Renee's brother Kenny was directly underneath Zach. Of course. When Renee was finishing up the ring, the small diamonds from my necklace fit perfectly in the Z, except for a few missing spots. Renee had kept some loose stones of Kenny's and two of his diamonds fit perfectly in the Z and completed the ring. I am sure that the two of them worked together to make that happen. I love my Z ring so much.

At the very end of that summer, my sister's friend Robin offered to do a reading for me. She is a very gifted medium.

> Robin: *Zach wants you to feel joy and not feel guilty about feeling joy, especially in front of people. Allow the grief, but keep working on feeling the joy. Find the balance. Spend time with the people who make you laugh out loud.*
>
> *He wants you to take a little break from the book and continue to find more balance.*
>
> *He is grateful that he can give you this advice and you will listen to it, and that he can help you from there. He is so grateful that you're so spiritual... so that not only did you*

put all of that spiritual stuff in his head which made it easier for him when he crossed over, but it also makes it easier for him to put that stuff in your head now.

I laughed. I said that now he has all the spiritual knowledge!

Robin: *Zach says that you should be very proud of yourself that you haven't been the kind of person to say to your boys, 'Don't leave me.' It is a testament to your strength and how good you've been that the two boys felt that they could go to Tampa and leave you after he died. Zach says, 'Thank you for letting all of my brothers still live their lives. You're wonderful, mom. Thanks for my whole life and for my childhood.'*

Zach's love always brings tears to my eyes. Once again, Zach knew exactly what I was feeling. As I began to heal and feel more joy, I felt self-conscious showing that to people. My son died, so wasn't I supposed to be sad for the rest of my life? I knew that wasn't true of course, but I had been feeling guilty showing joy in front of people, as if I was disrespecting Zach's memory. It truly helped to have Zach dispel that idea.

On September 17th, 2022, yet another tragedy struck. I got a call from my son Peter. He was crying and it was hard to understand him. One of his best friends, Carson Senfield, had been tragically killed in Tampa. Peter and his friends had gone to a game at University of South Carolina, but Carson had elected to stay behind with his fraternity to celebrate his 19th birthday. He died that day.

My first thought was that I wanted to fly to South Carolina immediately to be with Peter because I was really worried about him. He said that he and his friends were all together, they were okay, and they would take some time before they drove back to Tampa. I couldn't believe that he lost Carson just two years after losing his Zach. It was unimaginable. I couldn't believe that Carson was gone, another bright light gone from this earth.

It was almost too much to bear to think about my friends Bridget and

Darren, Carson's parents. It was too much to allow myself to think about their pain, for I knew exactly what that raw, piercing pain felt like. I went to their house to offer any support that I could. I knew from experience that Bridget would appreciate a hug from the only person who understood what she was going through. It was unbearable for me to see Carson's younger brother and sister, knowing how their lives were forever changed.

It was another huge loss for the Orchard Park community. Carson was a beautiful soul who was loved by everyone who knew him. Our whole family loved him. He and Peter had been friends since middle school. They grew up together. They went away to college together. Just a year ago, we had taken Carson with us to Florida for February break. He was like another younger brother to all of my boys.

Zach and Carson always had a special bond, even though Carson was seven years younger. Zach would pick Carson up for Peter's games and they would go together. They loved each other. Bridget said that Carson had taken it really hard when Zach died. One thing I knew for sure was that Zach was there for him when he crossed over, and took him under his wing. I have no doubt that they are doing great things together.

As with Zach, our community showed an unbelievable amount of love and support for the Senfields as they navigated through this tragedy, and the planning of a wake and funeral for their beloved son. I worried about my Peter as well. It has always been his way to try and uplift everyone around him. I worried that he wasn't processing this grief, but rather trying to be a support for everyone else. Still, I was grateful that Peter and Carson have an incredible group of friends that all pulled together to support one another, as well as the Senfield family.

I now knew why Zach had said to take a break from the book. I took a few steps backward when Carson died. It was like reliving Zach's death; the same time of year, the funeral at the same church, and seeing the excruciating pain on my friends' faces. My heart broke for them, and with them.

Since then, my friends Bridget and Darren have set up a foundation in Carson's memory, called the Carson Senfield Impact Foundation. They held an incredibly successful inaugural golf tournament, and I know they will do amazing things in Carson's honor. I know Carson is so proud of them.

CHAPTER THIRTY ONE

Our second annual Zachtoberfest was two weeks after Carson died. We obviously couldn't cancel because so many people had put so much work into it and we had so many donations of baskets and silent auction items, not to mention all of the people who already purchased tickets. And so we dedicated Zachtoberfest 2022 to our friend Carson and raffled a "Tampa" pennant with the proceeds going to his foundation. I know that Carson wouldn't have had it any other way.

It turned out to be even more uplifting than our first fundraiser. We held it at a different venue, The Wings Meeting Place in Orchard Park, and it was a perfect fit for us. There is both indoor and outdoor space, multiple bars, and two stages, so there are many niches where people can gather. The young people all gathered at the outside bar.

Once again, my sons' friends amazed me by their show of support. They came from all over the country. One of their friends said to me, "No matter where I am living, I will always come back for Zachtoberfest to support Zach and your family." It brought tears to my eyes. It was so good for Peter and Carson's friends who were there, just to be together.

Once again, Zachtoberfest was a fun night for all of us, and brought great healing to our family. Over 700 people came out for the event. My mom was able to come that year and she had a blast. It is such an enormous amount of work, but it is so worth it. Once again, our incredible committee (best team ever!) and all of our volunteers made it all possible. We raised $91,000 for Oishei Children's Hospital's Psychiatric clinic and OCD Program. It is impossible for me to thank every person who has donated or come to our fundraisers, so I will say it here: I am so incredibly grateful to every person who has contributed to the Zach Liberatore Foundation and to all of those who have attended our events. Our family is truly overwhelmed with gratitude.

Every year, Peter and I meet with the team from Oishei to talk about what our donation could support. The psychologists give us ideas and we actually have input toward the end result. It is one of my favorite days of the year. To date, the funds that Zach's foundation has raised have supported: Oishei Children's Hospital's Psychiatry TEMPO (Treatment for the Effective Management of Pediatric OCD) Clinic, transportation costs to increase access to quality care, community education on OCD, partnership with WNY school districts, Virtual Reality Exposure Therapy Headset, and partnership with Rogers Behavioral Health for residential treatment of OCD and related disorders.

The latter is my favorite. Rogers was the elusive treatment center that Zach could never get to, and where he had just gotten into when he died. The funds that we raised at our 2nd Zachtoberfest enabled five members of the Oishei OCD team to visit Rogers Behavioral Health Inpatient OCD program in Wisconsin to meet with members of their team for a day. They discussed program development and specific treatment approaches and began a collaborative relationship with their team, which will be helpful in facilitating future referrals from Oishei, which will in turn help the kids in WNY who struggle like Zach did. Nothing makes him prouder. Nothing makes me happier.

On Thanksgiving weekend, our family presented a check to the team at Oishei. It is another one of my favorite days. During the presentation, I received a text that another Orchard Park boy had died. He had played basketball with Christopher and I know his mom. She is one of the kindest and sweetest moms I know. Once again, it was too much to even think of another mom I knew going through that horror. I personally know FIVE moms who have lost a son since Zach died. It's too much.

Jillian had asked me a few months before why I wasn't teaching yoga for grief. She asked why I wasn't teaching people to heal themselves the way I had healed myself. I didn't have an answer. I had never thought of teaching a class for grief. When two more moms I knew had lost a child in the past two months, I knew that it was time. I wanted to help these moms in any way I could because I knew too well the excruciating pain they were in.

And so my grief yoga class was born. I put together all of the tools that I had used to heal myself after the loss of my Zach; breathing techniques, easy yoga poses, movement with sound, and I added sound bowls and a healing reiki meditation. I had purchased Paul Denniston's book, *Grief Yoga* and I loved some of his exercises so I added some of those. I added mantras and hand mudras and poses for heart chakra. Grief can get stuck anywhere in the body, but it especially affects the heart chakra.

I invited some of my friends who had experienced deep grief to my home studio for the first class. I knew that healing took place in that class, for them and for me. So I began teaching this class in the community. I posted about it on Facebook and Instagram and I had several friends, as well as complete strangers, offer their space for me to teach the class. I have also taught private classes for non profit organizations and I teach a monthly class sponsored by the town of Hamburg.

My friend Patti took my class and told me that she knew that the PUNT Foundation hosts a weekend remembrance retreat in Ellicottville, NY every year for parents who had lost a child to pediatric cancer and that it would be beautiful for me to teach my class there. I said, "I would be honored to teach my class there," but I didn't know how to make that happen. Literally the next day, I got a call from Terri Carbone who is on the board of the PUNT Foundation. Her son Nick had played football with Zach at Canisius. She told me how sorry she was about Zach, and that she and Nick had watched his funeral online together. And then she started telling me all about the weekend retreat in Ellicottville and she had heard about my class, and wanted to know if I would consider teaching grief yoga there.

I laughed at a photo of Zach as tears streamed down my face. How quickly Zach had stepped in! He heard me say that I would like to teach my class at this retreat, and I can just imagine him whispering in Terri's ear, "Mrs. Carbone, call my mom!" Of course he used a football mom to step in. It was a beautiful retreat and I was so honored to teach my class to a room full of bereaved parents. As I drove home, I was thinking how I would have loved to have had a remembrance weekend like that for my Zach. It was such a meaningful, healing experience for parents to honor their child. As far as I know, nothing like that is offered to parents who have lost a child to overdose, or suicide. Someday, I would love to offer grief retreats to all parents who have lost a child, or to anyone who is in deep grief.

The irony is, after a lifetime of trying to figure out what my "purpose" in life was, I finally found it. I feel that it is my responsibility to help people who are suffering with the loss of a loved one. I have had such amazing teachers, especially my Jillian, and I feel that it's my job to pass that knowledge along. I would not have wished for this path, for only in experiencing the loss of my beloved Zach did I learn how to heal myself step by step. Now I can pass on that knowledge to others. I especially feel very blessed that I am able to help bereaved parents. Of course, I would rather have Zach here and have a different life's purpose, but everything is exactly as it's supposed to be, or it wouldn't be. Still, I shed a tear as I wrote that.

I have heard that we carry the grief for the rest of our lives. I don't know if I believe that anymore. Grief gets "stuck" in our energy which can cause everything from depression to illness. As anyone who is in deep grief knows, it is so heavy. I think it's important to move it through our energy. Of course I will always carry pain over the loss of my Zach on earth and I will miss him every day for the rest of my life, but I no longer feel that deep grief within my body.

When I worked at moving grief through my energy physically (with breath and sound) and reframing my thoughts, I began to feel joy again. Slowly. Very slowly. Perhaps my greatest realization was that the happiness that we are always searching for is within us. After decades of reading that philosophy over and over, I finally understand what it means. Even though I'd read it a hundred times, it had to click. The simple truth is be it God, universal love, or divine energy that we are all searching for, it is within every one of us. Our soul, that light within us, is where we come from; it's what we truly are. Every one of us comes from the same source, that pure love energy. We are all connected. We hop into these earth bodies for awhile to learn and to grow our soul (I've heard it called "earth school") and then we go back home. Life is a blink, a dream. That happiness and joy that we are all always searching for is literally within us. The single best book that illustrated this for me was *The Greatest Secret*, by Rhonda Byrne. I suggest that you order this book today. Her simple techniques have been life changing for me.

There are several reasons why I wrote this book. First and foremost, I wanted to keep my Zach's name alive. All parents who lose a child worry that their child will be forgotten. I wanted to tell his story, especially for those who struggle like he did with mental illness and/or addiction, as well as their family members. There have been many dark times in my life when it helped to know that I wasn't the only one going through it. I know that Zach felt the same.

Perhaps my most important reason for writing this was that I hoped to help anyone who is in deep grief… in that overwhelmingly sad, empty, lonely place. Hopefully some of the tools that helped me can help others. I am not a psychologist or a guru, but I have experienced soul piercing grief. If just one person who reads this learns one helpful thing to help them heal, then it was worth all of my time and effort.

We are all just souls in bodies, who are having an experience on earth. We are made of energy and we have the ability to "shift" our energy. How can we do that?

- Start with breath. I feel that it is the quickest and easiest way to shift your energy. Try a breathing technique. Close your eyes, place your hands on your heart center and take twenty or thirty slow deep breaths. Or try the "Box technique"... inhale four counts, hold four counts, exhale four counts, hold four counts. Or try the 4-7-8 technique (my favorite). You can look it up online. Try whatever you're drawn to and whatever helps you.

- Movement. Move your body and get your energy flowing. Walk, run, exercise, or dance. Play your favorite song and dance. I cannot say enough about yoga. Don't cringe. You don't have to go to an hour and half power yoga class. Many years ago when I was doing my teacher training, our yoga philosophy teacher told us that it is more beneficial to do 15 minutes of yoga every day than a long class once or twice a week. I now completely agree with that. You can find many free "easy" short yoga classes online, or any kind of yoga you're searching for. Keep trying it until you find something that you like and that you will do. Yoga has always been the best way for me to get out of my head and into my body.

- Meditation. I know it sounds awful. And hard. It takes practice like anything else. For me, meditation is the single best way to connect with where we come from, to quiet the mind and connect with who we really are. There so many great free meditations online. There are apps that have meditations for beginners. I am a big fan of Master Sri Akarshana, The Honest Guys, and Great Meditation on YouTube. Keep trying until you find something you like and start with a very short meditation. A ten minute meditation each morning can change the tone of your day.

- Food. Food carries a vibration too. "Clean" eating raises your vibration; whole foods, fruits, vegetables, water, etc. are high vibrational. Meats, processed foods, and alcohol are low vibrational. (Don't hate me.) Food is a personal choice, but I know that cleaner eating helped me immensely when I was in deep grief.

- Thoughts. This is the biggest challenge for me. When I find my thoughts spiraling down into deep sadness and grief, I use a mantra to shift my energy; "I am so grateful that I had 24 years with my Zach on earth, and I am so grateful for the bond that we shared then, and still have." Another thing that helps when I catch myself having negative thoughts of any kind is mentally listing five things I am grateful for. Gratitude immediately raises our vibration.

These days, I am focused on my gratitude practice more than ever. Life always has it's challenges. After living together for 6 years, Keith and I mutually agreed to end our relationship. We will always maintain our friendship, but still it is another loss. I will always be grateful to him for his love for Zach and my boys, and for supporting me through the darkest of times, through unfathomable loss.

I am eternally grateful for the people who showed up for me and my family when Zach died, and continue to do so. Words cannot adequately express my gratitude to our family, friends, and our community for helping us navigate the unthinkable; just knowing the level of support that was there gave us strength.

I am so grateful for our Zach Liberatore Foundation, for the people who help us with our fundraisers, and all of the people who support it. It brings healing to me and Peter and our family. I will always have difficult days when I miss Zach so much it hurts, but when we find out about children and families that our foundation has helped, it softens the pain. I recently received a letter from a family whose 9 year old had been getting treatment for his severe OCD at the Oishei Clinic, but their insurance changed and his treatment was no longer covered. Our foundation was able to offset the cost for them so that he could continue treatment without a huge financial burden. His mom wrote,

At times we have felt like we are facing the 'invisible' battle that many people don't even know he's dealing with. However, when I remind myself about your foundation it helps, and not just financially. The reason is, it's telling me that we

Jennifer Liberatore

are facing this battle TOGETHER, that we DO have support, that others know what we are going through, that others know how difficult this can be, and they are here to help.

I feel so thankful that we are able to provide support like that to a family, and to help parents to not feel helpless, like we did. When I think of Zach's foundation helping that little 9 year old boy, I know with all of my heart that Zach intervened. I can feel his excitement that he is helping the kids who suffer like he did. I am truly grateful. Obviously not every parent who has lost a child has the desire or the support to start a foundation in their child's name, however any small positive act in your child's honor can make a difference. I read recently about a bereaved mom who goes to a local bakery on her son's birthday and pays for a birthday cake for another child. My friend Amy collects pantry donations for a local food bank every year on the day her son died. What lovely ways to spread love in their child's name.

Every day, my deepest gratitude is for my four sons. I am so honored that these extraordinary souls chose me to be their mom. They are my greatest blessings in this life. My pride and admiration for Christopher, Eric, and Peter is immeasurable. All three of them are kind, smart, hard-working, adventurous, strong, brave, amazing humans. They are filled with love. They gave me hope on my darkest days. They even dance with me.

My Christopher has always been my protector. After Zach died, he slid seamlessly into the role of oldest brother, always watching out for Eric and Peter. He lights up a room with his smile, energy, and infectious personality. He has a way of making anyone feel at ease in his presence. He makes everything fun.

My Eric is a free spirit with a heart of gold. He is compassionate, patient, non judgmental, and empathetic just like Zach was. He will do anything for anyone at anytime, especially his brothers. If they ask, he does. He never complains. About anything. I have always said that he is like sunshine.

My Peter is the most positive person I know. His enthusiasm for life (and everything!) is contagious. He intentionally and effortlessly uplifts everyone around him, including his brothers. He lives life to the fullest every single day. He has been a bubble of joy since the day he was born.

All three of them took the heartbreaking loss of their beloved Zach, and instead of it bringing them down, they used it to propel themselves forward. He wasn't just their big brother, he was their best friend. He was intertwined in the very fabric of their entire lives; no part of their lives had existed without him in it, until now. This tragedy could have broken them apart, but instead they choose to be even closer. On Christopher's last birthday, Eric and Peter went to Tampa to surprise him. I was sad that I couldn't be there. Then Eric's Lily sent me a video of the three of them, arms around each other in a huddle, jumping up and down, chanting. Anyone watching that video could feel the excitement, fun, and love between them. I have no doubt that Zach was right in the middle of them. Seeing that video was even better than being there.

After Zach's death, they could have easily fallen into sadness, self-pity, and anger, but they chose to move forward; living their lives with intent and purpose in their jobs, school, relationships, and friendships. They fight for their future. They live their lives with joy and meaning and I know that they do this for Zach, because he no longer can. There is no greater tribute to him. I am in awe of their strength and resilience.

My Zach. He was my dream come true from the first moment that I saw him. He was the one who made me a mom, my greatest job. He taught me kindness, compassion, patience, and empathy. He made me a better person. He was the strongest and bravest human I have ever known. He taught me by example to step out of my comfort zone of being private with my struggles, and instead to share my story and bare my pain, in the hope of helping someone else.

I miss him unbearably here on earth, but I know that he is not "gone" and I have not "lost" him. His radiant soul is always nearby. Some people think that Heaven is far away, somewhere beyond the clouds where our loved ones look down upon us, but Heaven is really just another dimension. Our loved ones are never far from us. Sometimes, I feel even closer to Zach than when he was alive, because now he is always with me. Our relationship did not end, it just changed. It is a new kind of relationship and our bond is stronger than ever.

In fact, when Zach was here on earth he missed out on a lot because of his mental health struggles, but now he doesn't miss out on anything. He is with me, his dad, his brothers, his baby sister, and everyone who loves him all of the time. He is at every family gathering, every birthday, every milestone, and he always will be. Whenever his brothers are together, he is with them. This I know for sure.

Melissa gave me a candle with a quote, *There are those who continue to light up the world long after they're gone.* That is surely Zach. He continues to help others, both here and on the other side. Sadly, another friend of his died recently and when I asked Jillian to send light to his family, she said, "Zach is assembling an army of angels." Of course he is. I can only imagine the amazing things that they are doing.

If you have lost a child, or you are in deep grief, just know that you will survive this, even though at times that may seem impossible. You will wonder how you will survive the pain, but you will. You may feel like you're surrounded by permeating darkness, like I did, but just know that the light IS still there. Be gentle with yourself. Healing takes time. Every day we have a choice to stay in the darkness or move toward the light. We get to choose how to live with our pain. We can allow our heartbreak to take us down or we can choose to be happy and live a meaningful life. It's not easy. It takes work, but it is so worth it and that is certainly what our loved ones want more than anything.

We recently held our third annual Zachtoberfest and it raised even more money and was even more uplifting than the past events, and I was so grateful, but I crashed so hard after it was over. Even though we are helping so many people in Zach's name, I would rather have Zach here. There will always be difficult days. The mama bear in me just misses her boy. A week later was the 3rd anniversary of Zach's death. It is always the hardest day of the year and my heart ached with missing him. I asked him to give me one bluejay. It is October and there aren't many bluejays around, but as I pulled into my sister's office, at that exact moment a bluejay flew right in front of my windshield in all of it's blue glory. I laughed. Zach letting me know he is right here.

Perhaps Winnie-the-Pooh said it best, *How lucky am I to have something that makes saying goodbye so hard.* Yes, how lucky was I to be loved by that boy. I know now that we didn't really say goodbye. I know that Zach wants me to be happy and to have a joyful life. I live for Zach now. The love that we had, and still have, is so powerful and we are spreading that love with everything that we do together in his name.

Love never dies.

ALBUM

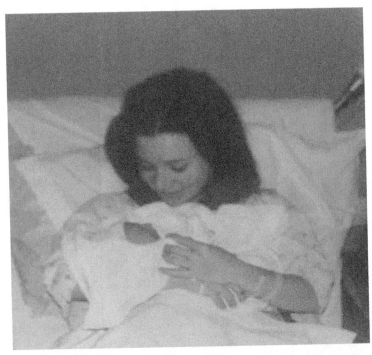

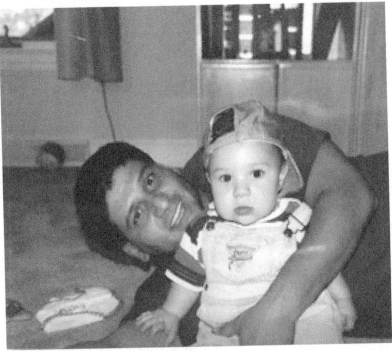

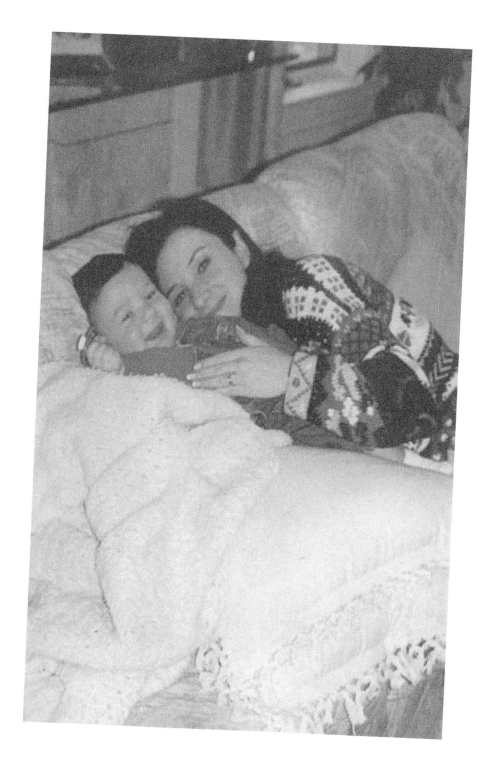

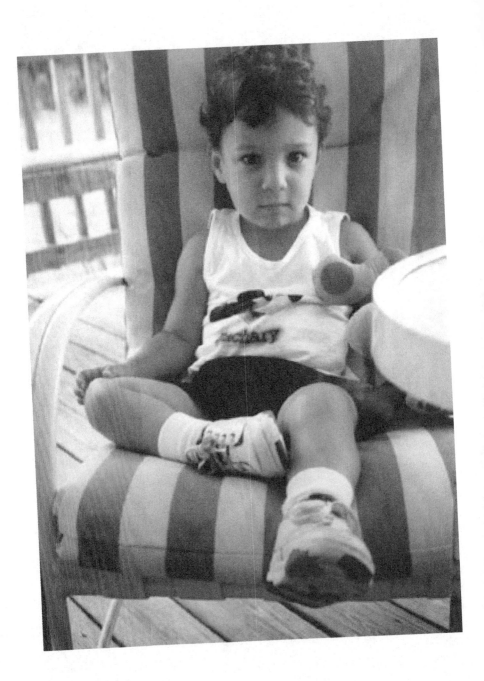

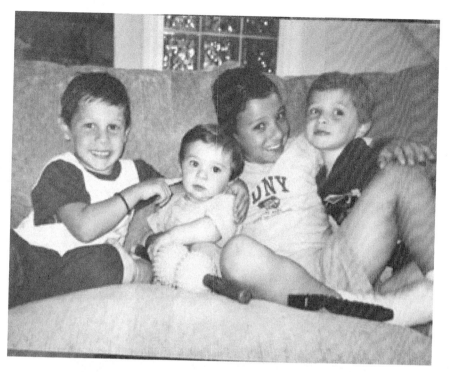

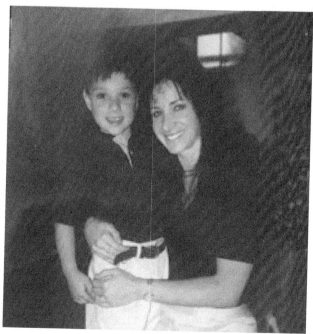

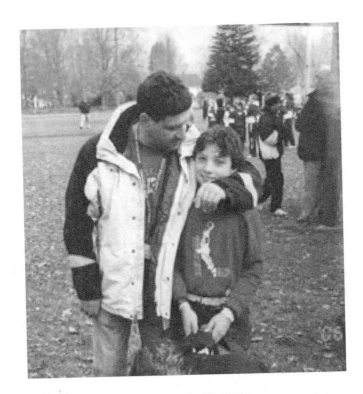

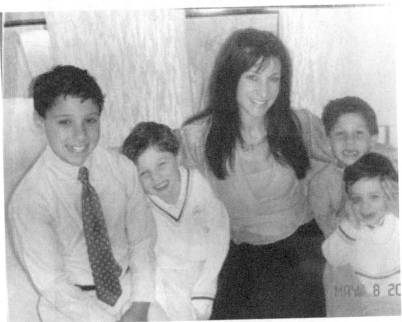

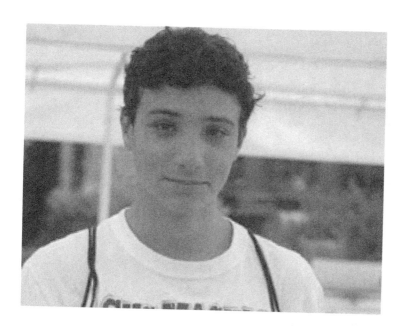

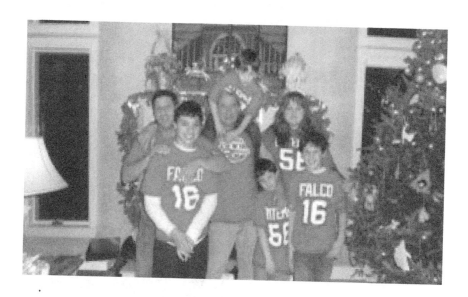

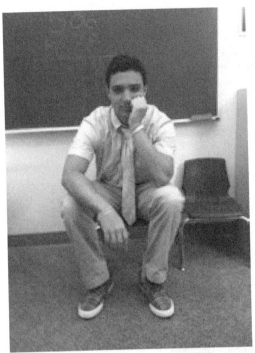

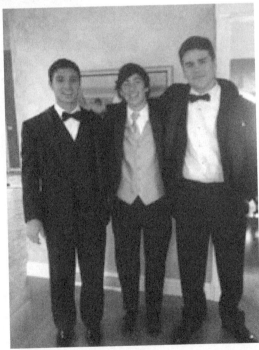

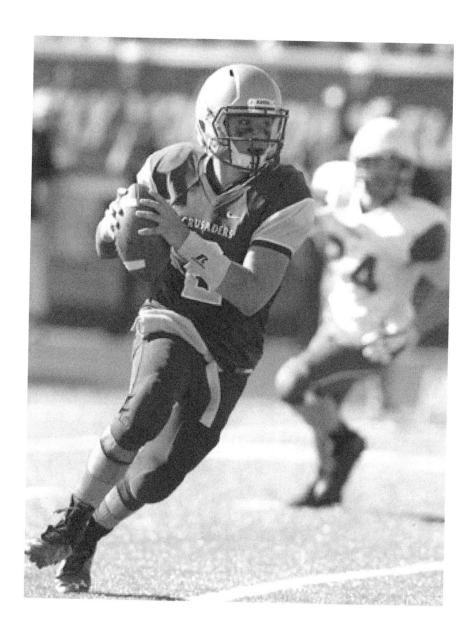

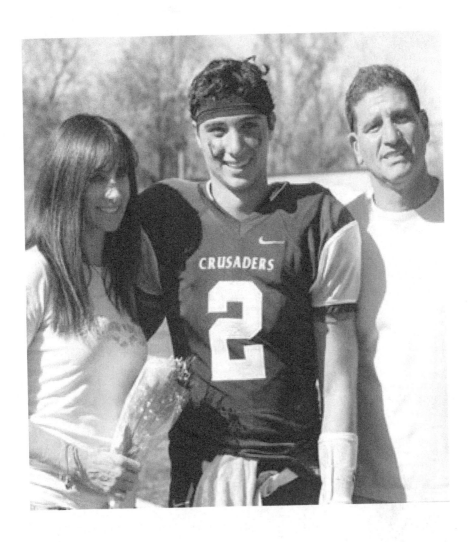

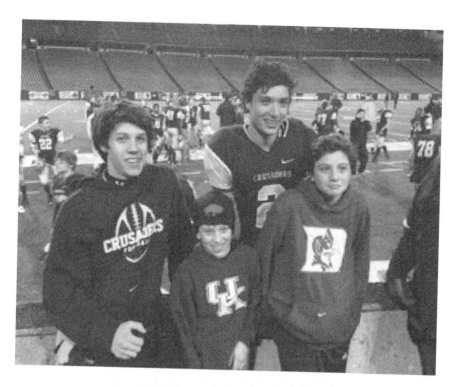

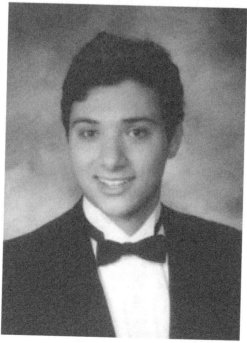

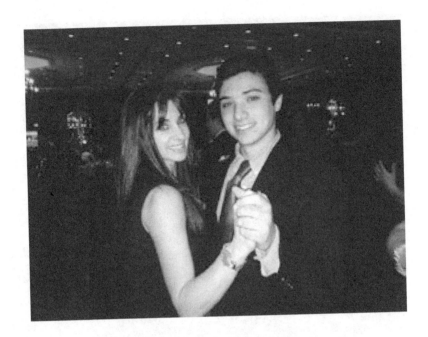

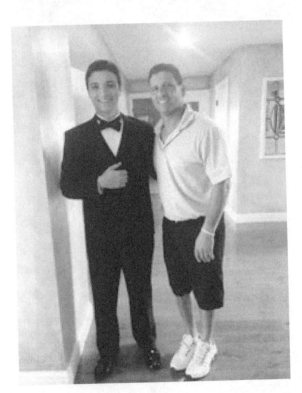

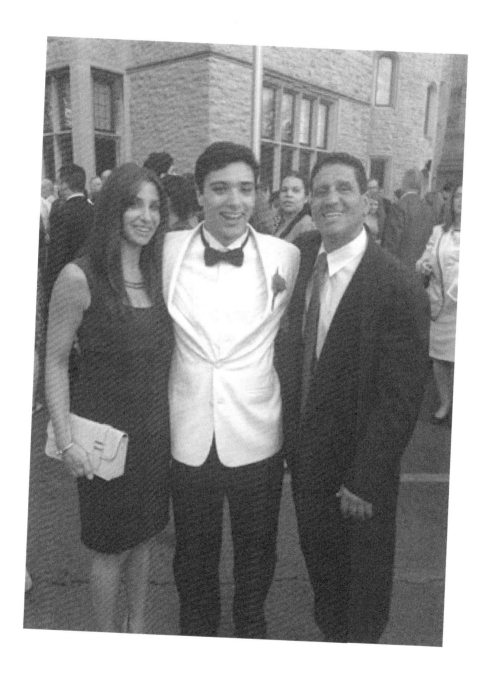

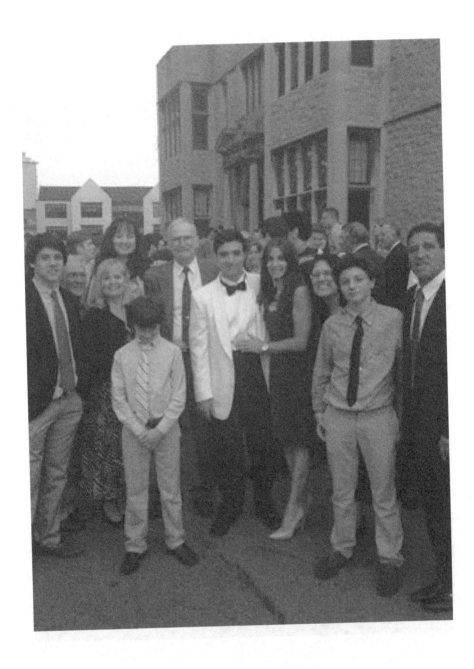

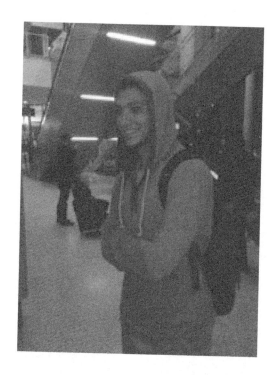

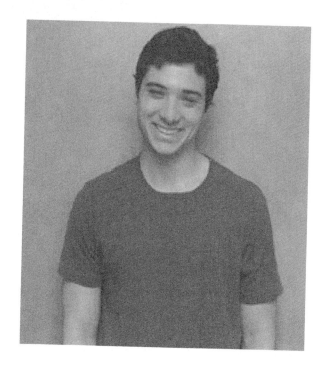

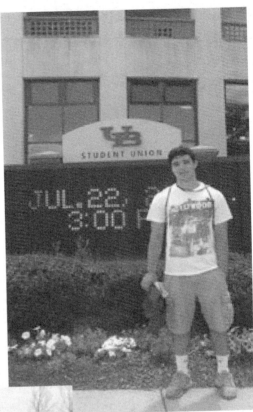

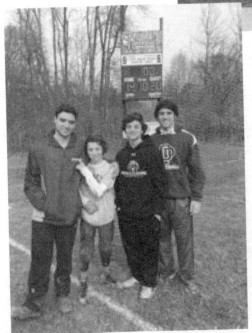

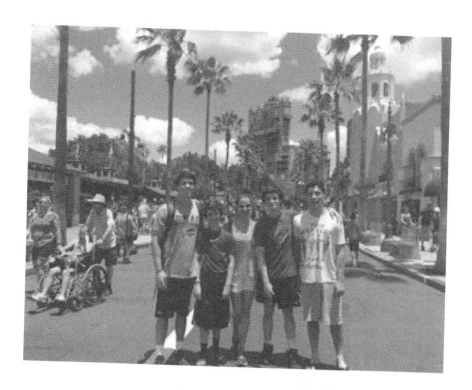

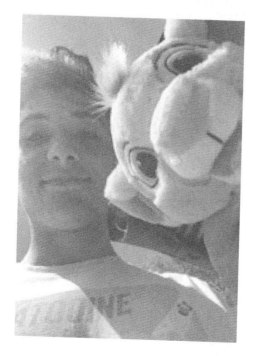

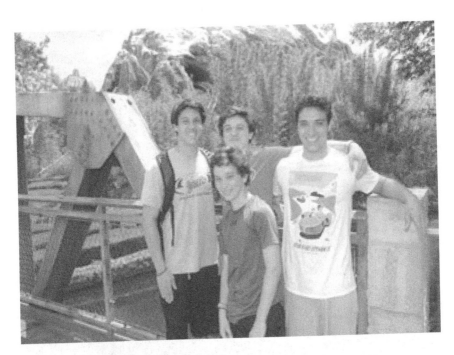

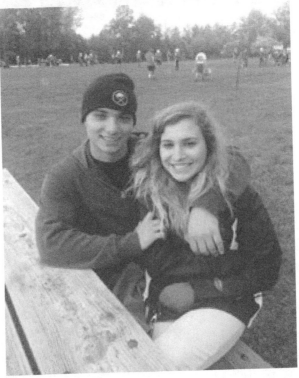

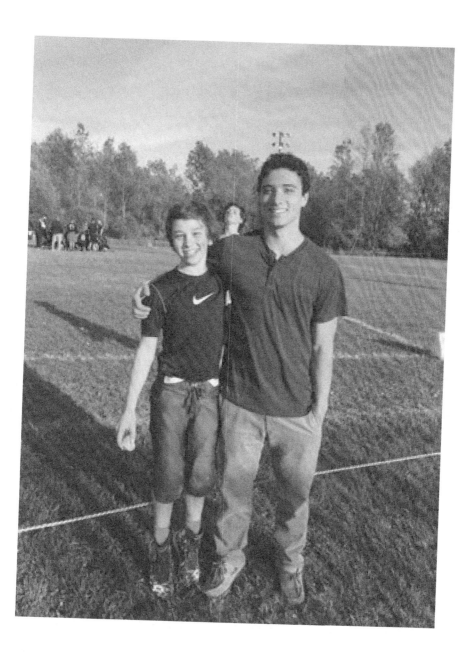

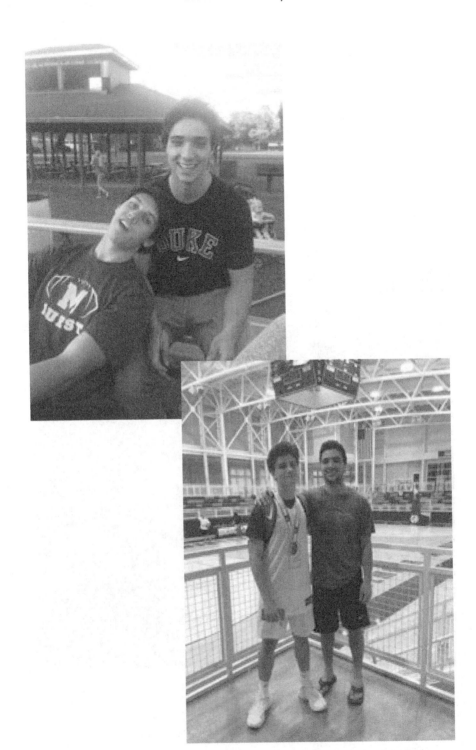

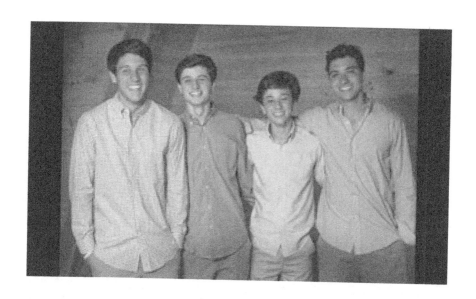

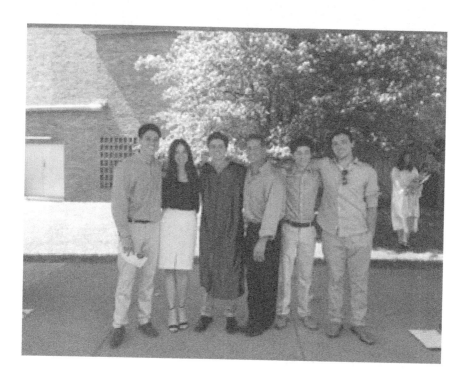

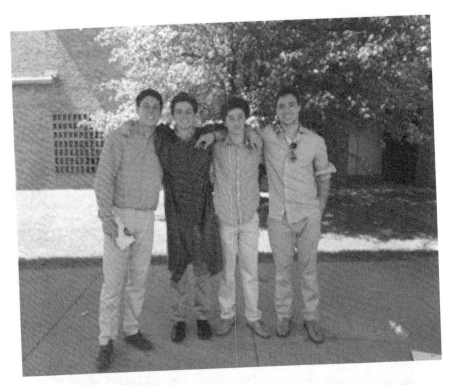

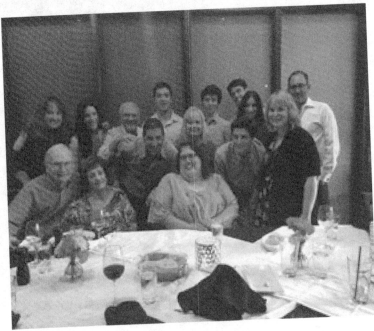

ïïïïïïﻹstop

Jennifer Liberatore

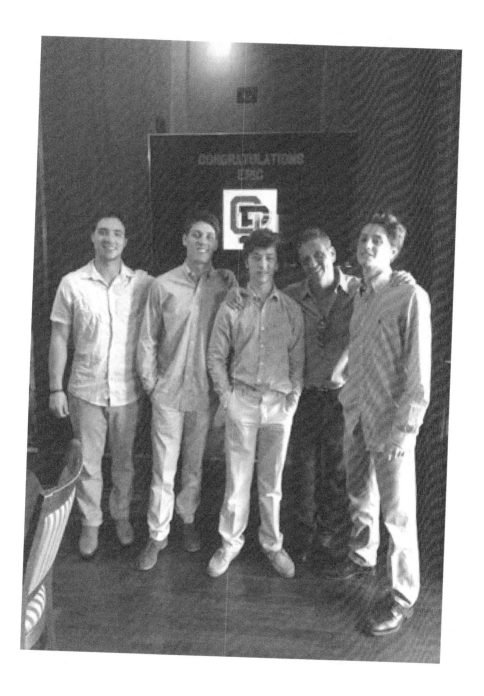

ïï

Jennifer Liberatore

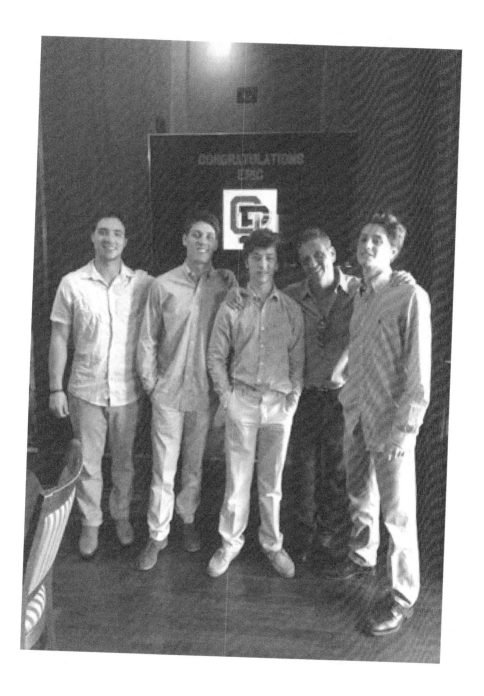

269

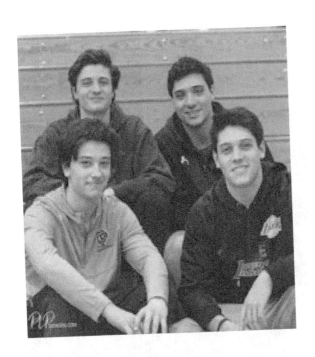

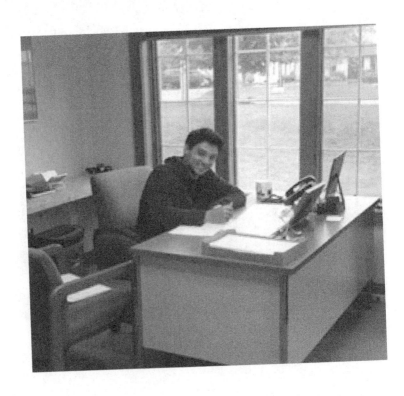

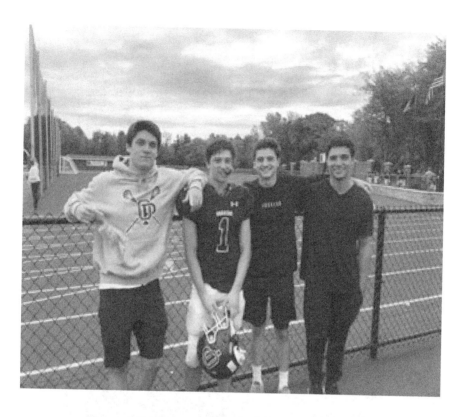

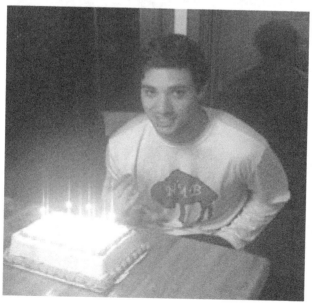

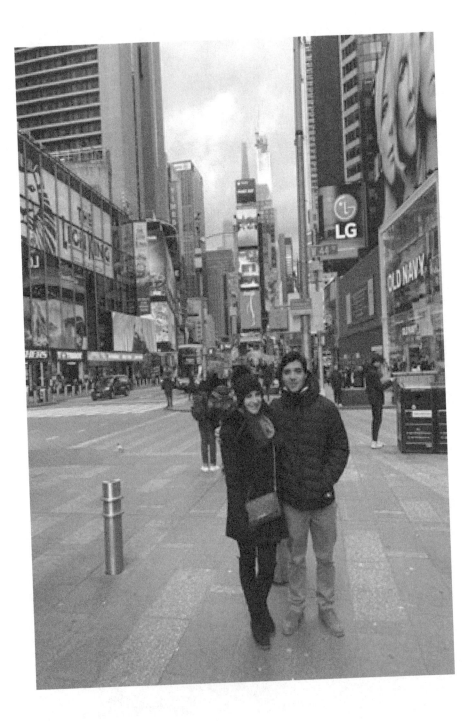

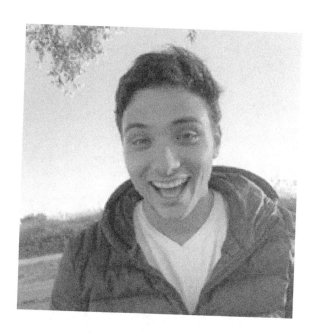

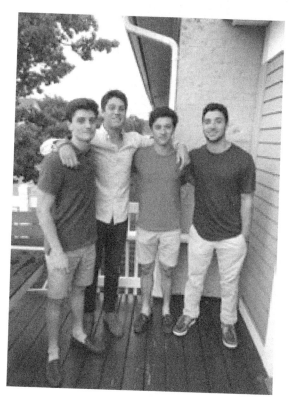

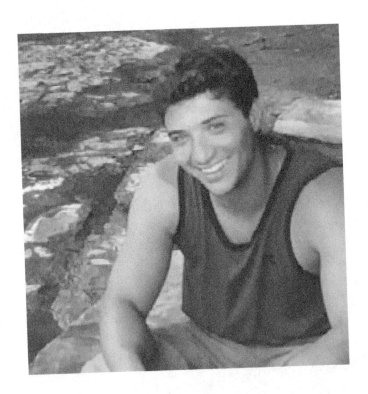

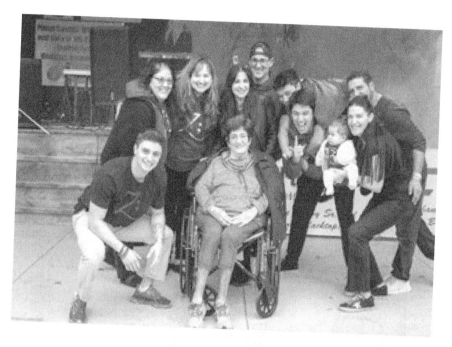

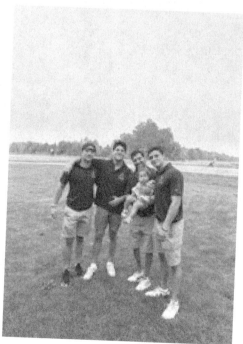

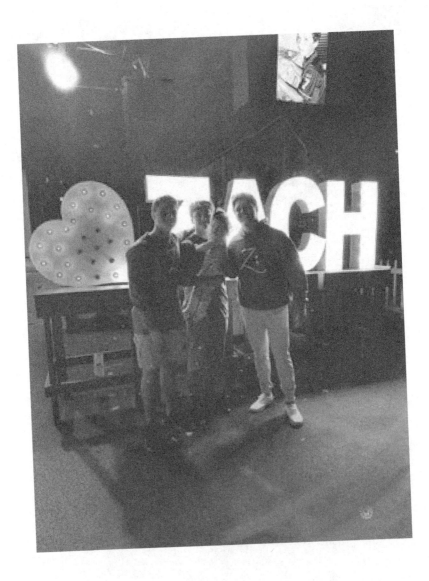

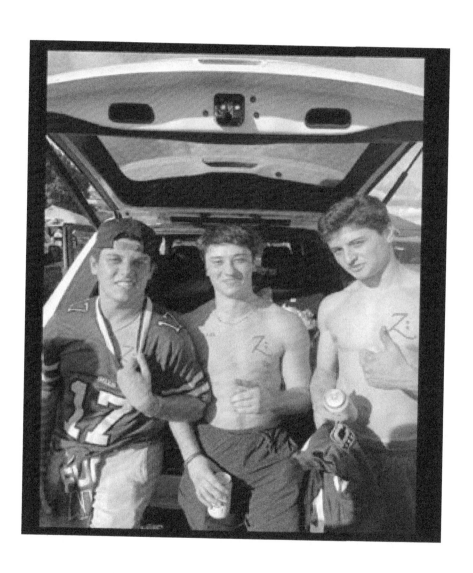

ACKNOWLEDGEMENTS

Special thanks to Jillian Greyse for sharing her light and wisdom with the world, and with me. I don't know how I would have gotten through the past few years without her. (jilliangreyse@gmail.com)

I'd also like to thank the spiritual counselors and mediums whose gifts to be able to connect with Zach greatly contributed to this book, as well as to my healing:

Krow Fischer (hereonearth.ca.), Peggy Lynch (lynchpeggy@aol.com), Leanne, and Robin.

I am so grateful to Zach's friends Morgan, Jenny, Raven, Drew and Danny for sharing their experiences of how Zach helped them, and for allowing me to share them.

A special thank you to Lily, for loving Zach, and for letting me include her in his story.

Thank you to Hannah Taylor (ahollowbone.com) for creating the beautiful cover design, and Patti (pattilooneyphotography.com) for the photos of Zach and my boys.

Thank you to my family and friends who support me in everything I do, especially my mom, Kerry, and Sue. Even when I had the crazy idea to write a book, every one of them was nothing but encouraging.

I am deeply grateful to Peter for going through this journey with me. He had no way of knowing that he would be dragged into it, as we spent hours in texts and calls going over the details of Zach's life. I also asked him to be the first to read the book, to approve of everything that I wrote about Zach. He read it in one morning and has been completely supportive.

Thank you to my sons Christopher, Eric and Peter for allowing me to write about their lives and our family.

And thank you to my Zach for encouraging me to share our story

Made in the USA
Middletown, DE
26 July 2024

57903145R00156